T0323105

QUALITATIVE RESEARCH METHODS FOR NURSES

Sara Miller McCune founded SAGE Publishing in 1965 to support the dissemination of usable knowledge and educate a global community. SAGE publishes more than 1000 journals and over 800 new books each year, spanning a wide range of subject areas. Our growing selection of library products includes archives, data, case studies and video. SAGE remains majority owned by our founder and after her lifetime will become owned by a charitable trust that secures the company's continued independence.

Los Angeles|London|New Delhi|Singapore|Washington DC|Melbourne

QUALITATIVE RESEARCH METHODS FOR NURSES

ROBERT DINGWALL
KAREN STANILAND

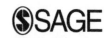

Los Angeles | London | New Delhi
Singapore | Washington DC | Melbourne

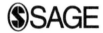

Los Angeles I London I New Delhi
Singapore I Washington DC I Melbourne

SAGE Publications Ltd
1 Oliver's Yard
55 City Road
London EC1Y 1SP

SAGE Publications Inc.
2455 Teller Road
Thousand Oaks, California 91320

SAGE Publications India Pvt Ltd
B 1/I 1 Mohan Cooperative Industrial Area
Mathura Road
New Delhi 110 044

SAGE Publications Asia-Pacific Pte Ltd
3 Church Street
#10-04 Samsung Hub
Singapore 049483

Editor: Jai Seaman
Assistant editor: Charlotte Bush
Assistant editor, digital: Sunita Patel
Production editor: Tanya Szwarnowska
Copyeditor: Solveig Gardner Servian
Proofreader: Brian McDowell
Indexer: Marie Selwood
Marketing manager: George Kimble
Cover design: Shaun Mercier
Typeset by: Cenveo Publisher Services
Printed in the UK

Library of Congress Control Number: 2020932584

British Library Cataloguing in Publication data

A catalogue record for this book is available from the British Library.

ISBN 978-1-4462-4875-1
ISBN 978-1-4462-4876-8 (pbk)

At SAGE we take sustainability seriously. Most of our products are printed in the UK using FSC papers and boards. When we print overseas we ensure sustainable papers are used as measured by the PREPS grading system. We undertake an annual audit to monitor our sustainability.

Contents

Author Biographies

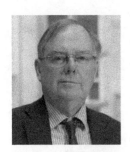 **Robert Dingwall** (RD) is a consulting sociologist and part-time Professor of Sociology at Nottingham Trent University. He has been researching and writing about issues in nursing history, policy and practice for more than forty years.

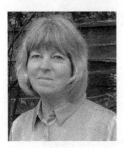 **Karen Staniland** (KS) was formerly a Senior Lecturer in Nursing at Salford University. After lengthy clinical experience in acute medical nursing, she trained as a nurse tutor and then as a researcher with a particular interest in quality and hospital organisation.

Online Resources

Discover your textbook's online resources!

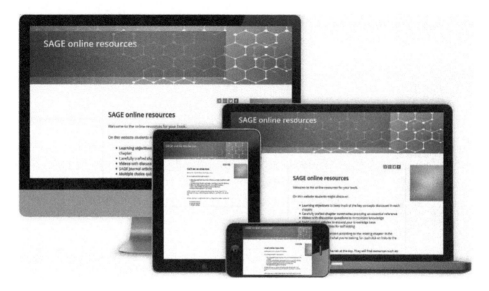

Qualitative Research Methods for Nurses is supported by a wealth of video resources. Find them at: https://study.sagepub.com/dingwallandstaniland.

Chapter introduction videos orientate you within the research process and set out the main topics and themes each chapter will cover.

Videos chosen by the authors from the SAGE Research Methods collection help you develop your understanding of key methods and techniques, such as interviews and conversation analysis.

Weblinks to **YouTube videos** vetted by the authors help you consolidate your knowledge of key concepts throughout the research process, from theory and picking a good research question to methods of data collection and writing up your research.

'Meet the author' videos introduce your guides to studying qualitative research methods and provide insight into how a researcher's journey unfolds in the real world.

Introduction

This is a practical and easy-to-use textbook for nursing students who are doing their first qualitative social research project. Our readers will also find it helpful in developing the flexible thinking that they need to deal with the clinical and organisational challenges presented by modern health care. We have written the book primarily as a basic text to be used by both pre-registration and qualified practitioners, doing qualitative research within the context of a first degree or a post-experience taught postgraduate course.

The context of health care and professional education is very different from that of ten years ago, when some currently used texts were originally published. Teaching methods have also changed – despite deteriorating staff/student ratios – with the adoption of more interactive approaches. Textbooks must support readers who have less tutorial time available to them.

The diversity of patients and practice settings continues to increase. Nursing students are also more diverse and often studying while working in clinical practice. They face issues in relation to methods and ethics that are additional to, or different from, those experienced by social scientists studying the same problems. This book explores the conflicts and tensions that can arise for professionals researching professional practice. It offers a clear analysis of the ethical and governance issues that surround qualitative research, and the ways these are shaped by the different impacts of employer, professional and university systems. We make extensive use of realistic case studies, often drawn from our own experiences of health care – shown as RD (Robert Dingwall) and KS (Karen Staniland) as professionals, researchers and users. The case studies are supplemented by self-assessment activities and questions to help you check your own analyses and understanding.

One important factor to mention here, is the 2020 COVID-19 pandemic (WHO, 2020), which had profound professional, social and personal challenging and unprecedented effects. We make some reference to this throughout the book and in one of the supporting videos on the website at https://study.sagepub.com/dingwallandstaniland. We know that this event will stimulate a great deal of new work in the research field and result in a very different landscape to what we have taken for granted in the past. We would urge you to write down any noticeable experience you were involved with before you get used to the 'new normal' and forget.

We have made three important, and quite deliberate, choices that distinguish this book from other qualitative methods textbooks that you might refer to:

1 **Many books on research methods for nurses focus quite narrowly on nursing and the use of these methods in nursing research.** We think that if nurses are researching the social, organisational and personal aspects of their profession and its practice, they are doing social research. This means that they should have the opportunity to draw on the full body of ideas and experience that have been developed when writing about societies, institutions and people. We hope you will come away from using this book with a sense of how what you do is building on mainstream traditions that go back more than two thousand years. Nursing research and nurse researchers may be relative newcomers but there is no reason why they should not draw on the full richness of this legacy.

2 **You will find people who think that qualitative methods are not scientific.** Some of these people think that only quantitative methods are scientific: others that qualitative methods are more like the knowledge of an artist, based on imagination and empathy. People who think that the term 'science' should be reserved for quantitative research sometimes quote Lord Kelvin, a distinguished 19th-century Scottish physicist, who asserted, in a public lecture in 1883, that 'when you cannot express it in numbers, your knowledge is of a meagre and unsatisfactory kind; it may be the beginning of knowledge, but you have scarcely in your thoughts advanced to the state of *Science*, whatever the matter may be' (Thompson, 1883). However, Kelvin also thought that heavier than air flight was impossible, that wireless communication had no use, and that X-rays were fraudulent … If you have stepped on to an aeroplane, logged on to a wi-fi network, or checked a patient X-ray, you might wonder whether thoughts like Kelvin's on quantification are any more valid.

   We think that science is a state of mind. It is about being systematic, sceptical and disinterested, at least while data are being collected and analysed. By this standard, we have no hesitation in describing what we offer in this book as a *scientific* education. In the same way, we do not put much weight on the claims that qualitative methods are distinctively about empathy. You will find that we emphasise collecting *evidence* by observing and recording what people say and do. Findings should be based on a systematic process of comparison and inference from data that can be made visible to, and checked by, other people.

3 **We have deliberately not said very much about the abstract theories within which qualitative methods may be embedded.** You will find a discussion of how theory is a way of bringing data together – but this is not the place to go into great detail about different schools of thought in sociology, anthropology, psychology or human geography and the ways in which they use qualitative methods. What we want to do is to help you get experience of doing qualitative research. If this excites you and you want to go further, you can learn more about these ways of thinking as your studies develop. If not, you will still have some useful experience and knowledge with which to evaluate other people's research reports that may, or may not, be helpful in your professional development and practice.

This approach complements more extensive reference textbooks or resources on qualitative health research – such as the handbook edited by Bourgeault, Dingwall and de Vries (2010) or Dingwall's (2008) collection of exemplary qualitative research in health care, which provide deeper treatment of specialist issues.

This book will get you started in developing projects that are directly focused on current challenges in nursing practice and the places where it happens. Qualitative research methods provide you with generic, transferable, tools that you can use in your everyday work to understand where patients are coming from, what is troubling them and their families, and how you can best use your professional skills and the resources of the organisation or network around you. Those same tools will also help you understand your workplace, the role of nursing within the provision of health care in contemporary societies, and the factors shaping the development and change of health care organisations, and the place of nursing within them.

HOW TO USE THIS BOOK

We have broken up the text with the following learning features:

- Learning Outcomes
- Definitions
- Case Study Scenarios
- Self-assessment Activities
- Reflections on Practice
- Critical Thinking Exercises
- Freeing our Imagination
- Key Point(s)
- Video Support
- Chapter summary points
- Further reading

These will help you to develop your independent learning skills. You will have noticed that we have included the term 'Freeing our imagination': rather than just imitating what you see around you, we want to encourage you to develop alternatives that might break rules or get out of the ruts of conventional thinking. This approach was suggested by Becker and Leibovici (available at http://howardsbecker.com/images/book-covers/becker-leibovici-exercises.pdf).

At various points, we have suggested further reading and references. You should look at some of these to broaden your learning, although we also encourage you to read beyond them. The book is not designed to be read in a single session. Each chapter takes you forward one step in the development, design and execution of a research project. If you are using this book to help with a dissertation, for example, studying in a group that agrees to read a chapter at a time, and discuss it, may be a good way to move forward. The group does not have to meet face to face – maybe you could set something up on social media?

VISUAL ASPECTS

One of the teaching methods that has changed is the greater reference to, and integrated use of, visual materials for students who learn more effectively in this way. Where possible, we have either created video resources or directly linked to existing materials, which you can access via the book's online resources (https://study.sagepub.com/dingwallandstaniland). You can also find further material yourself by searching on YouTube, although bear in mind that the quality and credibility of these videos can be variable.

We hope that you enjoy the book, and good luck with your studies!

1

What is Research and Why Does it Matter?

Learning Outcomes

At the end of this chapter you will be able to:

- Discuss what research is and why it is important in health care
- Outline the development of research and theory in health care
- Summarise the relationship between research, theory and practice
- Review your professional and organisational expectations for research
- Summarise why ethical research matters

When you first encounter research, you might easily think that it is something exotic, carried out by distinct kinds of people who work in special kinds of organisations. There is some truth in this: as with many activities, some people develop particular expertise and focus on research as their career. If you stop and think for a minute, though, you should realise that everybody does some sort of research every day. Any time you read a newspaper, visit a website, ask someone for advice, whether face to face or on social media, or look around a room to see what is happening, you are doing research. You may do this just because you are curious and want to be better-informed about the world you live in. Often however, you are doing it because you have some sort of practical problem that you want to solve. What car should I buy? Where should I go on holiday? Where do I look for a bus timetable? We usually carry out these investigations in a simple fashion, using our ordinary skills at everyday living. However, even a basic training in research methods can help us to do such inquiries more effectively.

> **Definition**
>
> **Research** is a word that describes the many different approaches that people use to investigate problems. In a professional context, like health care, 'research' is a particularly systematic inquiry directed towards increasing individual or shared knowledge about a topic.

THE PROBLEM OF TRADITION

Research skills matter because they help us define the object of our search more precisely, identify what information would be relevant, assemble this quickly and systematically, and evaluate its quality as a basis for making a decision. These skills are increasingly important in contemporary nursing practice. In the past, much nursing care was delivered with very little investigation. Students were trained to assume that every possible problem had been solved in the way that 'things had always been done'. If you had a problem, this was because you had not learned that tradition well enough. There could never be a problem with the tradition itself.

Nursing tradition, for example, used to dictate that hospital beds were made in a specific way. You may be too young to remember the old Nightingale wards where beds were made with blankets and sheets, arranged to produce very precise 'hospital corners'. Some ward sisters and matrons would even measure that the edges of the sheets dropped the same distance on every bed! Nursing tasks were delegated on the basis of seniority to meet the obvious 'physical' care needs of the patients. One of the students in Kath Melia's classic qualitative study of nurse education in the late 1970s described the very end of this system:

> If you are a staff nurse you don't get a bedpan, if you are a third year, you don't get a bedpan – if you've got no stripes [i.e. a first-year student], you've got the bedpan! (Melia, 1987: 42)

The following extract, from a blog by Julie Vuolo (1987), describes her experiences of nursing in the 1970s:

> The ward was run by a Sister who was close (not close enough some might say) to retirement. She was German and 'old school'. She purred after the consultants and shouted at the junior doctors. She rang the visiting bell in the visitors' faces if they didn't leave exactly on time and she insisted that all the bed wheels faced in the same direction so that the ward looked tidy. She was also well known for hiding in the large walk-in linen cupboard during a cardiac arrest call (fortunately rare in our area) and for delegating all difficult tasks to her very accomplished deputy.
>
> The main ward was set out in the traditional 'Nightingale' fashion, with beds lined up either side and a table and some waist-high storage cupboards in the centre. This was in the days when

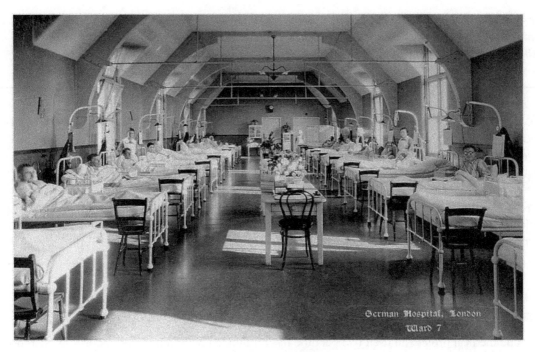

Figure 1.1   A ward set out in 'Nightingale' fashion

visitors could still bring in flowers which would then be left in vases in various stages of decay until we went and sorted them out. Although against hospital regulations, Sister insisted that we use spray wax polish on all the hard surfaces to keep the ward looking and smelling clean. We were supposed to use the damp dusting method as this was 'proven' to keep dust and dirt under control so we kept a spray can of polish and some dusters hidden on the ward to use when the supervisors weren't around. Despite Sister's antipathy toward damp dusting she did allow the ward floor to be polished with the buffing machine, a big heavy machine with a mind of its own that took some mastering. Though difficult to control, the floors were left looking beautiful, slippery as ice mind, but beautiful all the same. (Vuolo, 1987, reprinted with permission)

Today, we would say that the ward was full of harmful bacteria, slip-and-trip hazards, and indifferent to the psychological wellbeing of patients. Think about all the adverse incident reports you might be asked to fill in!

If you are interested, Walsh and Ford (1989) describe more of the rituals and myths that used to abound in hospital wards. How many of these are still hampering progress in nursing care? At the same time, you might also want to think about the potential benefits of ritual. After all, it does mean that you don't have to think about every challenge every time you encounter it. Perhaps it is sometimes important as a source of psychological relief or a way to disengage emotionally from a difficult situation, as Menzies (1960) suggested in a study of ward life in the late 1950s.

———————— FREEING OUR IMAGINATION ————————

Would you have dared to challenge that ward sister? If so, how would you have gone about it?

You might be amused by this account, but you should also see some reasons to be concerned. Was this ward clean? Was it a safe place to work? Was it good for patients to marginalise their friends and relatives? Maybe the sister's behaviour was actually based on some long-forgotten theory or since-discredited research. This had become so embedded in her practice that the original reasoning had been forgotten – we may never know!

The limitations of 'uncritically' relying on tradition within nursing and other health professions began to be recognised in the 1950s. Why did this model fail? Four important reasons are:

- The medical profession itself had become less influenced by tradition and incorporated a more questioning approach from research scientists, whose work was built on challenging established knowledge.
- Clinical work moved out of the stable and controlled settings of hospitals, which changed little between the mid-19th and mid-20th centuries, into more fluid community environments.
- Patient populations became more diverse as people lived longer with the diseases, disorders and disabilities of a more affluent, ageing and multi-cultural society.
- Greater diversity within the medical and nursing professions meant that former relationships of class, gender and ethnicity were less effective as a basis of hierarchy and authority within health care. This increasingly rested on expertise rather than status – what you knew rather than who you were.

This transition has not been an easy journey and is not yet complete. There is always a tension between stability and change in people's work. Organisations and professions try to establish practice routines and rituals because these can be efficient and make the work manageable. You cannot question everything all the time, especially in clinical emergencies. However, if you never question anything, then you never change anything. You gradually fail to deliver what your patients or clients need at a cost that a society can afford.

Key Point

Why does research matter? Because it is a critical source of innovation to serve the changing needs of patients and society.

RESEARCH, THEORY AND PRACTICE

In most natural and social sciences, research forms part of a circuit that connects practice with theory (see Figure 1.2)

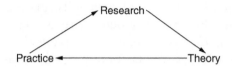

Figure 1.2   Circuit of research, practice and theory

Problems in practice prompt questions for research, which develops theory that can then inform practice. Sometimes, research can also be stimulated by problems with a theory, when findings are inconsistent with each other, or with what the theory predicted.

Key Point

Research can start out as a response to problems that can often lead to practical benefits.

- *Immediate practical problems* – Where should I go on holiday?
- *Theoretical problems* – What does care mean?
- *Curiosity-driven problems* – Curiosity is the key of everything, not just science. How/why does/doesn't this work? What is it that is going on here?

To do this work, researchers need to develop some distinctive language. Think about those mornings when you wake up and feel somewhat unwell. Your head hurts, your joints ache, maybe you have a cough and a runny nose. Your temperature may be up a little. You have to tell your partner or housemates that you do not feel like getting out of bed and going to work today. What words do you use? A 'cold'? A touch of 'flu'? A bit of a 'chill'? 'Man flu'? If your first language is not English, perhaps you have some other words to describe this experience. This vague language is fine for everyday purposes. It is enough to communicate how you feel to the people immediately around you. Of course, they may not agree with your description. Perhaps they will accuse you of drinking too much the night before and trying to make excuses for a hangover. The point is that the language works in this context.

Suppose, however, that you are working as a clinician or a scientist. Now you need to be much more precise. You need to use words that connect these experiences to specific causes and provide a basis for research to develop treatments or to prescribe appropriate medications. Most of these symptoms are caused by viruses, but sometimes they can be caused by bacteria. If they are bacterial, they can probably be treated by antibiotics; if they are not, these drugs will have no effect and the prescription just increases the likelihood of resistant strains developing, which is not in anyone's interest. Both bacteria and viruses come in a variety of species or types. Although there are fewer options for anti-viral therapy, as a clinician it is still helpful to know what you are dealing with, to inform treatment and prognosis. So, we find different language being introduced: 'influenza', a potentially serious illness caused by a specific group of viruses, which are moderately susceptible to a small number of drugs; 'common cold', a minor illness caused by a different and larger group of viruses, for which there is no effective treatment other than symptom relief. These new words are detached from the everyday experience of sufferers, but they can now be used among clinicians and scientists to be sure that they are all talking among themselves about the same thing. The words can also travel across the borders between different disciplines, languages and areas of practice.

Of course, these various processes of translation between *everyday* and *scientific* language are not completely straightforward, and even scientific language use involves quite a lot of negotiation and uncertainty. These translation processes are a topic for social science researchers, who have developed their own language for talking about them. In the same way, people who do research in nursing have developed a specific language, or borrowed one from other social sciences, that allows them to look at a particular context or issue as a case study. The immediate findings can be translated into a more abstract form that allows them to be transported to other locations that provide other cases. At each site, the abstract language is converted back into questions about 'what is going on here?' that help the researcher, or practitioner, to understand what they are seeing and hearing. This abstract language is what people who do social research, including nursing research, call *theory*. Because theory is a way of summarising or generalising from specific cases, there is always some room for arguments about how best to carry out the processes of translation and conversion. In this book, we shall not say a great deal about the different kinds of theory associated with qualitative methods, and the reasons why some people might prefer one to another. If you go further in research, though, you will need to learn more about them.

> **Definition**
>
> **Theory** is a way to take the findings of research projects and turn them into more general statements. These can then be translated back to the specific circumstances of new practice problems. This means that the language of theory is always rather abstract. If it were not, it could not do its job of taking knowledge from one context to another.

HOW DOES THEORY WORK? AN EXAMPLE

Nursing is often described as a 'caring' profession (see Figure 1.3). If you are working as a nurse, then, it might seem logical that you would know or pick up what 'care', 'caring', 'tender loving care

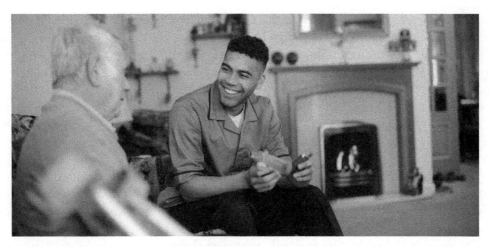

Figure 1.3   Nursing: a 'caring' profession

Credit: iStock.com/sturti

(TLC)', 'all care' or 'basic care' means. You might think this is obvious. However, you could test that assumption by writing some short notes in answer to the questions below.

CRITICAL THINKING EXERCISE

What does 'care' mean?

- Is there an official definition of 'caring' where I work?
- Is this expressed in a caring framework intended to guide my practice?
- How do the definition and the framework match up with what caring actually means to people like me when we are doing it?
- How do we learn what counts as caring in this context?
- Does everybody working in our team have the same ideas about what caring is and how to do it?
- Does caring mean the same thing to patients and their relatives as it does to us?
- Do we understand 'caring' in the same way as our nursing colleagues in the next ward, or the care home down the road, or in the community, working in the next village or neighbourhood?
- Are some people (women, gay men, members of specific ethnic groups?) thought to be more naturally gifted as carers than others (heterosexual men, members of other ethnic groups)?

When you have written these notes, try to think about 'care' in other contexts. What does it mean in other health care settings you have worked in, or experienced as a patient? What does it mean in your family? What does it mean among your group of friends? What did it mean when you were at school? Have you seen any advertising or marketing for companies that claim to 'care' for their customers – what do they mean by this?

How did you do? Let's consider a couple of points. If you have found that there is not a definition of caring where you work, how do you know everybody knows what it is? How do you deliver 'care' to the same standard? If care means different things to different members of staff, then standards will obviously vary.

You will probably find that people are using the same word in many ways with different meanings. You can try to develop a way of classifying these meanings – care[1], care[2], care[3] and so on. This is the beginning of developing a *theory* of care. As you advance this, you can see how it helps you to notice things about other contexts.

We shall come back to this in more detail in the next chapter.

SCIENCE AND ETHICS

If you have developed a theory of care based on your findings about what it means to different groups, you can evaluate it in two ways. One question is about whether it accurately captures the meaning that care has. The other is whether that meaning is morally or ethically acceptable. The criteria for the second judgement come from a different way of thinking. This tries to picture an ideal world and then to think about how the real world could be made to look like that. You could call this a *philosophy* of care. It is also important because debates about ideals are another way to challenge the standards of practice. If you only look at what is happening, you may settle for what you can achieve rather than aspiring to do better. However, if you only ever think in ideal terms, you may never recognise that real life is about compromises. Some ethicists think patient autonomy is very important, for instance, so that patients should be able to choose any treatment they think might benefit them. However, if you are working in a system where health care is paid for by taxes or compulsory insurance, you might ask whether this is fair to the people who are footing the bill. Should they have to pay for other people to receive treatments that do not have a proven benefit or will only deliver a small benefit at great cost? Is there another ethical principle here? The aspiration to treat patients as autonomous is a worthy one – but you might not want to pretend to them that it is always possible.

Qualitative methods are sometimes thought to be especially useful in informing ethical debates. However, it is always important to remember that there is a big difference between understanding the world as it is and thinking about how it might be better. These objectives should not be confused. Ethical conclusions rarely follow directly from research evidence: this can often be used to justify a variety of policies and practices. The choice between them may reflect an ethical position you already hold, but while you are carrying out the research, a scientific approach means that your first obligation is to your data. As we said in the Introduction, science is a state of mind – systematic, sceptical and disinterested – not a set of practices for measuring and counting.

> ## Key Point
>
> Research matters because it develops theory that makes it easier for knowledge to move from one situation to another.
>
> Research matters because it allows *theory* and *practice* to be evaluated against moral or ethical *ideals* – and for those ideals to be tested against the real world.
>
> Research tests whether 'the way we have always done things ...' is 'the best way of doing them'.

WHAT IS KNOWLEDGE?

You may remember that we mentioned earlier how research can describe any systematic way of gathering information. Only information that we are sure about can properly be called 'knowledge'. The study of knowledge is a point where social science research meets the area of philosophy called *epistemology*.

Epistemology is the branch of philosophy concerned with the nature and scope of knowledge. It is sometimes also referred to as 'theory of knowledge'.

Definition

———————————— VIDEO SUPPORT ————————————

If you find epistemology a difficult concept to understand, try watching Kent Löfgren's classic video, *What is Epistemology? Introduction to the Word and Concept*. You can access the video by visiting this book's online resources: https://study.sagepub.com/dingwallandstaniland.

Common sense and science

Throughout our lives we 'learn' and 'remember' to do many everyday things. We have learned, for instance, how to use technology from the moment we wake up and look at the clock or phone to tell the time, to turning on the radio, making our first cup of tea or coffee and travelling to work. We know how to do these things because we have absorbed information from all around us: conversations with other people, reading, television, social media, the Internet – the list is endless.

We have a lot of confidence in this *tacit* or *common-sense knowledge* because it works so consistently. We take it for granted that when we press a button, the radio will turn on. We do not constantly question all these things: life is too short. It is only when something fails to perform as we expected that we start to reflect on our tacit knowledge: the radio fails to come on – Is the battery flat? Has there been a power cut? Has a fuse blown? Has the button stopped making a good contact because of wear and tear? We can work through these possibilities to decide whether we need to spend a few pence on a new fuse or battery or several pounds on a new radio.

Even in work settings in health care, a lot of knowledge is tacit. Professionals assume that readings from patient monitors are reliable because they mostly are. This becomes a problem when a machine fails. RD had a near-miss during a hospital episode with septic shock when a monitor gave false readings that implied fluid infusions were failing to correct a low blood pressure. Inappropriate clinical interventions were only avoided when an experienced doctor took a pulse manually and recognised that its strength was not consistent with the monitor readings. Everyone else just 'knew' that the machine was correct.

We need to think about how we get our knowledge, what our knowledge is based on, how widely it might be applicable and how closely it is likely to correspond to reality. Some examples of how we acquire knowledge, can be by:

- *Authority* – knowledge given by somebody you trust, such as a parent (but it does not mean that it is necessarily true – parents used to tell children babies were found under gooseberry bushes!).
- *Experience* – repeatedly using a practical skill, like inserting a cannula, for example.
- *Tradition* – learning by asking how something was previously done.
- *Revelation* – reading the sacred texts of a faith group or experiencing a direct contact with a supernatural source.
- *Logic* – constructing forms of arguments and testing their validity according to formal, public and shared rules for correct reasoning.
- *Empirical* – based on objective facts established by explicit and transparent investigative processes.

Key Point

Common sense or tacit knowledge is not easily shared. Although we all use it, we cannot necessarily say what it is. It consists of beliefs, ideals, values, schemata and mental models which we mostly take for granted and do not think about. While difficult to articulate, tacit knowledge shapes the ordinary ways in which we perceive the world and perform routine, everyday tasks and actions. People are often not aware of the tacit knowledge they possess or how it can be valuable to others.

——————— FREEING OUR IMAGINATION ———————

In everyday life we do not generally question everything all the time: it can be very annoying when we do. You can test this for yourself.

For example, an American sociologist called Harold Garfinkel devised a series of experiments to reveal how much tacit knowledge we took for granted in our every-day lives. One of these involves asking other people to explain what they mean in conversation. Instead of replying 'I'm fine' when someone asks 'How are you today', try answering 'What do you mean, 'how am I'?' Keep asking them to explain their answers and see how long it takes for the other person to get very cross! Daily life works because we can trust that the people we meet and work with share a lot of tacit knowledge with us. The world around us seems stable and predictable and we can approach it with confidence.

However, there are other kinds of knowledge that arise from systematically doubting things that we ordinarily take for granted. This was the basis of the creation of the natural and social sciences in the 17th and 18th centuries. For example, in 1500, everyone in Europe 'knew' that the Sun revolved around the Earth. By 1800, it was universally accepted, at least among people who had had some schooling, that the Earth revolved around the Sun. This transformation came about because several astronomers found anomalies in their observations that undermined their confidence in what had been taken for granted (like your radio not working) and led them to search for an explanation. That search produced a new way of thinking that was consistently supported by other observations and became accepted as knowledge.

The success of this model led others to adopt what was called *radical doubt*, where every element of tacit knowledge could, in principle, be challenged. Very often, the results showed that 'what everyone knew to be true' was wrong. Partial and inaccurate observations, or a reluctance to move away from traditional sources of authority like the Bible, had entrenched misleading pictures of the world.

In 1654, James Ussher, Archbishop of Armagh, had calculated that, according to his reading of the Bible, the world had been created on the evening preceding Sunday, October 23, 4004BC. By 1788, James Hutton, a Scottish physician, was arguing, based on his own geological observations, that the Earth had to be much older than this, although his work was not fully accepted until the 1830s. The resulting conflicts between faith in authority and scientific scepticism continue.

In practice, these categories often interact with each other. Returning to the previous example, when your radio fails and you investigate the cause, you are acting like a scientist, testing out various possible explanations so you can re-create a stable feature of your environment – that your radio works. In laboratories, scientists often rely on instruments that have been designed to create shortcuts, so they do not have to doubt everything (we shall say more about this in Chapter 8). Many measuring tools are like that: a chemist trusts that a spectrometer works in just the same way as you trust your radio. To go back to a previous example, everyone on the ward 'knew' that RD's blood pressure monitor could be trusted. When Harold Garfinkel had his students press their friends and family to keep explaining what they meant, he was treating common sense (everyone knows how to answer the question 'How are you today') as an object for scientific inquiry – what happens when someone does not produce the expected answer? Nevertheless, it is important to know what kind of knowledge you are using at any particular moment, so you know how much to trust it and what to do if it does not work.

Key Point

We have, then, two kinds of knowledge:

- One, which we often call common sense, is *tacit*, an unquestioned background to everyday, routine activities. This often seems intuitive, although it is, of course, something we have learned throughout our lives – from other people, from books or other media, or from our own experiences.
- The other, which we often call *scientific*, is based on scepticism and doubt, where we have deliberately set out to question something that seems obvious, like the Sun revolving around the Earth or that increasing the price of a product or service means that people will buy less of it. Scepticism and doubt can be applied equally in the natural and the social sciences.

CRITICAL THINKING EXERCISE

When you train to be a health professional in a particular field, you acquire both scientific and tacit knowledge in that field. Rycroft-Malone et al. (2004) suggest that professional knowledge is derived from the following four sources:

- Knowledge from research evidence.
- Knowledge from clinical experience.
- Knowledge from patients, clients and carers.
- Knowledge from local context and environment.

Can you identify which of these sources of knowledge are likely to be tacit and which are likely to be scientific?

NURSING RESEARCH AND NURSING THEORY

It is important to note that *nursing* research and theory has not always been developed in a systematic way. Historically, both were caught up in a project to invent a body of expert knowledge unique to nursing that would improve the profession's status and bargaining power in relation to other health care occupations and the wider society (Traynor, 1999; McCrae, 2012). As Dingwall (1974) had pointed out, nursing research often seemed to be undertaken more as a symbol of the profession's aspirations rather than as a systematic contribution to investigating and solving clinical, organisational or interpersonal challenges for practising nurses. Traynor (1999) suggested the failure to develop a credible evidence base recognised as meeting wider scientific standards had undermined the profession's case for the value of its practice.

> An **evidence base for practice** can come in many forms, but in essence it involves combining individual clinical experience and expertise with the best available guidance from systematic research, wherever this originates.

Definition

French (2002) also criticised nursing research for this attempt to produce a special kind of knowledge, rather than benchmarking this against basic disciplines. Nurses working on microbiological questions, for example, would look to each other rather than to the general field of microbiology to assess the quality of their contributions. Similarly, nurses using psychology, anthropology or sociology to inform their research would not go back to the standards of those disciplines but would pass them through a professional filter. There was, however, nothing distinctive about a 'nursing way of knowing' other than the selective use of this knowledge to address nursing's specific interests and practice challenges. Nursing was not taking part in the creation of a general pool of knowledge from which it could draw for its own purposes as required. The failure to engage with the wider natural and social scientific communities made it harder for nursing to absorb new knowledge from outside: studies of how organisations innovate has shown how important it is for them to be doing their own research to be able to understand and integrate other people's (Cohen and Levinthal, 1990). This is why we often refer in this book to studies from outside nursing – to help you make use of knowledge from other fields to improve research and innovation within nursing.

The consequences of seeing theory and research mainly as a way to achieve professional status could be seen in two ways. First, clinical practitioners made little use of either theory or research to inform their everyday work (Bircumshaw, 1990). Second, the profession lacked a good way to defend the importance of basing practice in research and theory against the anti-intellectualism of some commentators: journalists, politicians, and some nurses, repeatedly assert that a caring heart is more important than intellectual ability. It is also often highly gendered – women are assumed to care more than men.

At its best, this scepticism reflects a belief that *altruism* alone is the way to provide the most appropriate and humane care (Melia, 1987; Witz, 1992).

Definition

Altruism is an attitude or way of behaving marked by unselfish concern for the welfare of others.

At its worst, this scepticism reflects a serious misunderstanding of the complex technical and social challenges of much modern nursing, and the need for practice to have a strong natural and social scientific foundation (Dingwall and Allen, 2001; Allen, 2014a). This was underlined during the COVID-19 pandemic where nurses were able rapidly to build on this foundation and acquire the sophisticated skills necessary to manage breathing support.

REFLECT ON PRACTICE

We shall say more about Allen's work later, but you might find it useful to look quickly at the website from her study of the 'invisible work' of nurses to see how she has built a theory, *care trajectory management*, out of her observations of 'what nurses actually do all day': https://theinvisibleworkofnurses.co.uk/.

PROFESSIONAL AND ORGANISATIONAL EXPECTATIONS

Up to this point we have discussed why research might be important mainly at an individual level – why *you* should want to understand research to help develop your own clinical judgement and decision making and for the benefit of *your* patients, clients or service users. This is something that all health professionals should learn throughout their training (Ashley and Stamp, 2014; Cappelletti et al., 2014; Cranley et al., 2009). It is always the most important reason why nurses should want to be aware of and to keep up with research. However, nurses have a licence from a regulatory body to practise and are almost invariably employed by some kind of organisation. It is, then, also important to understand the expectations of regulators and employers, if only to stay out of trouble in getting and keeping a job. In the UK, for example, this means the requirements of the Nursing and Midwifery Council, together with the policies of the health departments of the various national governments. (In practice, the health departments tend to work together at a UK level on professional issues.) These constitute the framework within which health and social care organisations employ and manage their nursing staff.

UK health departments have consistently emphasised their commitment to improving the quality of patient care through research and the use of its findings. As long ago as 1972, the Briggs Report asserted that nursing should become a research-based profession. This was widely misunderstood as saying that every nurse should be doing research alongside their clinical duties: the report actually said that this should be the sort of specialist role that we described at the beginning of this chapter. However, it did call for 'a sense of the need for research [to] become part of the mental equipment of every practising nurse or midwife' (p. 108). Every nurse could give their patients better care if they understood how to use research reports to improve their practice – and this meant that every nurse had to understand something about what research involved. This message was repeated in the Department of Health's (1999) policy statement on nursing, *Making a Difference: Strengthening the Nursing, Midwifery and Health Visiting Contribution to Health and Social Care* (we have added the emphasis in all the following quotes):

> Practice needs to be evidence-based. Research evidence will be rigorously assessed and made assessable. Nurses, midwives and health visitors need **better research appraisal skills** to translate research findings into practice. (Department of Health, 1999: 44).

The Government's response to the recommendations in Front Line Care: The Report of the Prime Minister's Commission on the Future of Nursing and Midwifery in England (Department of Health, 2011: 16) stated:

> It is essential that practice, education and research should be integrated. Clinical and research career pathways for nurses and midwives should be planned more effectively between NHS, other health providers and universities through strong clinical leadership locally. Commissioners will need to **base their decisions** about models of care, service delivery and health outcomes **on evidence**.

The Department of Health's (2012) Developing the Role of the Clinical Academic Researcher in the Nursing, Midwifery and Allied Health Professions declared:

> This strategy will support the Government's aim to improve people's health outcomes and the experiences they have of their care by developing the best research professionals. High-quality research must be generated and translated at the point of care to facilitate improvement. The clinical academic workforce will be instrumental in ensuring **diffusion and spread** of best practice and innovation.

The updated 2015 Nursing and Midwifery Council's *Code* (2018a: 9) presents the *professional standards* that *nurses, midwives and nursing associates* must uphold in order to be registered to practise in the UK:

6 Always practise in line with the best available evidence. To achieve this, you must:

6.1 make sure that any information or advice given **is evidence-based** including information relating to using any health and care products or services. In other countries, such as America and Australia the same themes, principles and barriers to developing skills in and integrating research to practice apply, albeit in slightly different formats and stages of development.

You should already be familiar with the fourth edition of the Nursing and Midwifery Council's (2018b) *Future Nurse: Standards of Proficiency for Registered Nurses*, which refers to research and research awareness in Platform 1 (1.7).

Similar statements can be found in other countries. The Nursing and Midwifery Board of Australia's (2018) *Midwife Standards for Practice* Standard 1 promotes health and wellbeing through evidence-based midwifery practice:

The midwife supports women's wellbeing by providing safe, quality midwifery health care **using the best available evidence and resources**, with the principles of primary health care and cultural safety as foundations for practice.

In the USA, The National Council of State Boards of Nursing (NCSBN) (2015) Research section states:

NCSBN conducts cutting-edge, award-winning research that supports evidence-based regulatory decisions for patient safety and public protection.

WHY DOES RESEARCH MATTER?

- There are explicit organisational and professional expectations that every nurse will be aware of the knowledge base for their work and make critical and appropriate use of it in their practice.
- It is a way to demonstrate that nursing is meeting the expectations of the people who pay for its work that this is being carried out to the highest standards.
- As a nurse, *you* are personally and professionally accountable for your actions and care, so it is essential to be up to date with the current evidence base for practice which is based on relevant research. This includes being able to critically appraise new research in your field and to consider whether it is good enough to influence your practice.

CHAPTER SUMMARY POINTS

This chapter has discussed what research is and why it is important in nursing. We have briefly outlined the development of research and theory, and summarised the relationship between research, theory and practice, mentioning ethics. We hope you now appreciate the influence of nursing tradition and the importance of questioning this. You should also be able to review your professional and organisational expectations for research and to summarise *why research matters*.

This chapter has begun to give you some food for thought. First, to encourage you to think carefully about what might be expected of you as a professional practitioner. Second, to start questioning *'What is it that is going on here?'* in your own practice as the beginning of a research journey.

FURTHER READING

To help with the context for this chapter, you could read some of the classic early research in nursing published by the Royal College of Nursing, such as:

Boore, J.R.P. (1978) *Prescription for Recovery*. London: Royal College of Nursing.

Hayward, J. (1975) *Information – A Prescription Against Pain*. London: Royal College of Nursing.

Stockwell, F. (1972) *The Unpopular Patient*. London: Royal College of Nursing.

McCrae (2012) has looked at the literature on theory and nursing models since the 1950s and discussed their value in the context of evidence-based practice and multidisciplinary health care. For many writers, theory has mainly been part of the process of seeking to improve the *professional* status of nursing as much as, if not more than, improving the quality of care:

McCrae, N. (2012) 'Whither nursing models? The value of nursing theory in the context of evidence-based practice and multidisciplinary health care', *Journal of Advanced Nursing*, 68(1): 222–9. https://onlinelibrary.wiley.com/doi/abs/10.1111/j.1365-2648.2011.05821.x (accessed 24/2/20).

2

Theory and Methodology

Learning Outcomes

At the end of this chapter you will be able to:

- Identify different research problem types
- Outline the challenges in defining practical problems
- Outline the challenges in defining theoretical problems
- Outline the challenges of defining curiosity problems
- Define methodology and method
- Describe three basic qualitative methods
- Explain how inductive and deductive reasoning influence theory development

In the previous chapter we introduced the idea that the research started out as a response to problems that can often lead to practical benefits.

These problems might be:

- *Immediate practical problems* – Where should I go on holiday?
- *Theoretical problems* – What does care mean?
- *Curiosity-driven problems* – What is happening here? You don't really know what you will find but you hope to achieve a better understanding of something.

> ## Key Point
>
> Research aims to change your state of knowledge about a problem. You may not be able to *solve* the problem, but it should, at least, help you to *understand* and *manage* it better.

However, if research is going to be really useful, you should be able to pass its findings on to other people and apply it to other problems without having to re-do everything from scratch. If there is no way to share or transfer knowledge, then you will waste a lot of time reinventing wheels. This is where theory comes in. Because this is a book about qualitative research methods, we are not going to discuss particular *theories* in detail here. We shall mention some of those that are particularly associated with qualitative research as we go along. However, we think that it is really important that you do not develop the impression that research methods are just a set of technical skills.

This chapter may appear abstract and you might wonder what it has to do with research. Can't we just get on and tell you how to do interviews or focus groups or observations? Our response is that if you do not understand what these skills are based on, you cannot evaluate your own work and join the results to other people's in ways that make them more useful for everybody. This understanding is also important for reviewing other people's work, to decide how valid it might be and whether you should take account of it in your own research or practice. You may find it helpful to come back to this chapter again when you have read more of the book, but stick with us for now.

> ## Key Point
>
> Knowledge moves on by being translated into a more general language, and then translated back again in a new context. You do not need to learn how to read a bus timetable, or use a bus app, every time you want this information. You have learned the skills so you can look at a document or a screen with a particular format and pick out the relevant details. You do this more or less automatically because it is such a regular and simple task that the underlying knowledge has become common sense – fixed and tacit.

As we saw in the first chapter, many elements of health care have involved traditions that reflected long-forgotten theories which had become embedded in practice. Taking flowers to people in hospital, for example, goes back to the time when disease was thought to be transmitted by miasmas (bad smells or bad air). Repeated observations that certain diseases seemed to be associated with people who gave off bad smells, or lived in evil-smelling neighbourhoods, were linked together to create *miasmatic theory*, that the smells were causing, or at least transmitting, the diseases. Using this theory, doctors and nurses reasoned that surrounding sick people with nice smells and fresh air would promote their recovery. During the 19th century, the discovery of bacteria (known then as 'germs') gradually led to the replacement of miasmatic theory by *germ theory*, which saw miasmas as simply an indicator of conditions in which harmful bacteria thrived. This change did not happen quickly – there is an echo of miasmatic theory in the way the smell of the polish favoured by Julie Vuolo's ward sister (in the previous chapter) signalled the absence of infection. However, nice smells do not guarantee an absence of disease-causing organisms: flower water has been shown to be a rich source of unwanted bacteria. In UK hospitals at least, flowers now tend to be excluded from hospital rooms. You can see further debate about this with a simple internet search of 'flowers in hospital'.

PRACTICAL PROBLEMS

It is quite difficult to explain tacit knowledge because it is such a matter of habit. Look at how RD thought about a problem when he went on an architectural tour of a new hospital in Chicago in the early 2000s. The hospital architect, who was leading the tour, explained that his original design had two sinks in each single room – one for patients to wash in and one for staff undertaking clinical procedures. However, his research with this layout found that staff often failed to wash their hands because they were not sure which sink to use. RD translated this as showing that the staff had a problem with using their tacit knowledge to classify the sinks: should they use the (hypothetically) 'clean' patient's sink or the 'dirty' clinical sink? As a result, they often used neither.

The architect's solution was a design change to provide an extra sink just inside the doorway for staff to use as they left, before they went to their next patient. The number of sinks now matched the tacit classification of 'clean' and 'dirty' tasks used by the hospital staff. However, RD had also learned that the staff did not seem to classify tasks as simply 'clean' and 'dirty' but used three categories: 'clean', 'a bit dirty but clean enough', and 'really, really dirty'. This example shows how he turned a specific observation about sinks into knowledge that could be used elsewhere by developing a theoretical language – a set of abstract categories that are sufficiently generalisable to be applied in other contexts.

Key Point

It is important to stress that RD's categories are social not microbiological. A sink may be socially 'clean' but microbiologically 'dirty'. The difference is important in understanding how cross-infections occur.

Now try this activity for yourself.

CASE STUDY SCENARIO

Think about the continuous struggle to improve hand-washing in health care. Ask someone who is not a health care worker to tell you (not show you) how they wash their hands. Can they describe this process? Can you tell them (not show them) how to wash their hands in a way that will remove more bacteria?

You have probably found this quite hard because neither you nor the other person have quite the right words to describe this process. You do not have an abstract language to talk about what is going on. One of the challenges for people who are trying to improve hand safety in hospitals is to create this language so that they can compare what happens in different places or different departments. Photographs or video clips of hand washing may *illustrate* differences, but these differences can only be *discussed* and *explained* through words. Microbiologists can test the skin surfaces and map the bacteria that they find on people's hands using well-established language: this bacterium is called *E.coli* and that bacterium is called *c. difficile*. Giving the bacterium a name links it to other observations about its distribution and about measures that have been found to be effective in controlling or eliminating it. Social scientists could try to classify styles of hand washing and give them names so anyone can recognise instances of these categories and develop appropriate organisational or training responses.

CRITICAL THINKING EXERCISE

You could put 'hand washing demonstration in health care setting' into You-Tube and see how many actual demonstrations you can find. It is interesting too to see if the commentary is linked to the demonstration.
   Give it a go!

THEORETICAL PROBLEMS

If one of the things we do with research is to investigate tacit knowledge, another is to evaluate the results of applying previously established scientific knowledge or theory. You are likely to find this in dealing with questions about the best way to organise professional work, whether in a hospital or a community.

Social scientists have been writing about this problem for more than one hundred years so there is a great deal of research and theory about professions, work and organisations. You might think this is quite long enough to answer the question. In fact, it turns out that the question is a very complex one because the best answer depends on the context and what the organisation is being asked to achieve.

Key Point

If you look at health care, you will find the following tensions around what professionals and organisations are expected to deliver:

- *Equality vs Equity* – should everybody be treated exactly the same or should they be treated differently to reflect their different needs and expectations?
- *Personalized care vs Collective benefit* – should every patient get everything they want, regardless of the cost, or should the allocation of resources be constrained by the ward's budget and the likelihood that a patient will actually benefit from being given what they want?
- *Continuity of care vs Expertise and specialism* – should every patient be treated as far as possible by the same individual professionals or should their clinical needs be broken down so that each can be dealt with by the best available specialist?
- *Quality assurance vs Quality of care* – should resources be committed to management systems that attempt to ensure that frontline care is efficient, effective, equitable and humane or just given to the frontline staff to use as they think best?
- *Professional autonomy vs Organisational governance* – should professionals simply allocate resources for the benefit of the individual patients in their immediate care or should they take some account of the general interests of the hospital, or the health care system, or the interests of the people who pay tax or insurance fees to cover the costs?

You may be able to add some more but it should already be clear why it is difficult, if not impossible, to devise a way of organising work that will always resolve all of these tensions at the same time to everyone's satisfaction. Nevertheless, we can make certain predictions about the consequences of a design that favours some goals rather than others as demonstrated in the next critical reflection.

REFLECT ON PRACTICE

If hospitals are rewarded (or punished) for achieving (or missing) financial tar-gets, then they will tend to work in ways that prioritise resource management over clinical outcomes, which makes them vulnerable to criticism for the death of patients.

If they favour clinical over financial outcomes, they are likely to be criticised for wasting other people's money, whether from taxes or insurance.

Most real organisations must find compromises between theoretical ideals – we shall say more about these later when we introduce the notion of an ideal type.

CURIOSITY PROBLEMS

Finally, we have curiosity-driven research – sometimes called 'blue-skies' research. You might won-der why people should be given time and resources to do research just because they are curious about how something works – some people think all research should have an immediate practical objective, especially in an applied field like health care. However, this kind of research is often the most productive and innovative precisely because it is not driven by a pre-existing problem. In fact, we often have to ask a lot of questions about a problem and turn it inside out before we can do research on it – which really irritates people who think the problem is obvious.

In the late 1930s, some US hospital patients were being treated with such high doses of opiates that doctors would describe them as physically dependent on the drugs. However, when the drugs were withdrawn, these patients did not show the desperation of addicts in the community trying to fight the distress of this experience, and to recover the euphoria produced by the opiates. Social scientists' curiosity about this behaviour led them to discover the importance of the way patients understand their sensations of their own body. Patients only craved more opiates if they realised that the withdrawal symptoms were caused by the lack of the drugs rather than the natural course of recovery from the injuries being treated.

Alfred Lindesmith (1965), a sociologist who is particularly associated with this work, had already been studying addicts in the community in Chicago. His discovery was also primed by theoretical ideas that were widespread within sociology at the time. Essentially, these said that people acted on the basis of their perceptions of the world rather than on their response to objective reality: as another Chicago sociologist, W.I. Thomas, put it, 'if men define situations as real, they are real in their consequences' (Thomas and Thomas, 1928: 572)[1]. Today, we might refer to 'people' rather

---

[1] If you want to know why his wife, Dorothy Swaine Thomas, does not share the credit for this observation, look at Merton (1995), where she explicitly denies any part in it.

than 'men', although some feminist writers have observed that women may find it harder to make their definitions have real consequences! In the next paragraph, which is less often quoted, the authors also go on to accept that people cannot just define situations in any way they want to. Would you like to fly from London to Rome with a pilot who defined the Alps as molehills instead of mountains? You could, then, say that Lindesmith was prepared to study this problem – but it still needed the moment of curiosity to create the opportunity.

You may be wondering why we have included this old example. What is important is that Lindesmith's work has stimulated a long line of research on how people *learned* to experience the sensations produced by various psychoactive drugs as pleasurable, or the absence of these drugs as a source of pain, discomfort or distress. This pointed to the importance of the *contexts* in which they were introduced to drugs and what shaped these. Some practitioners and policymakers have been led to question whether many of the bad experiences that seemed to result from addiction were actually produced by public policies that prevented the legal supply of affordable drugs of reliable and consistent quality, so that addicts had to associate with criminals.

Thinking in this way also helps us to understand the effects of some legal drugs like steroids and, indeed, the benefits of advance information for helping patients recover from surgery (Hayward, 1975). Remember the quote classically used in nurse education by McCaffery and Beebe (1989), which echoes Thomas's words:

> Pain is whatever the experiencing person says it is, existing whenever the experiencing person says it does.

If people are prepared for post-operative pain and adequately believed and treated for it, they seem to manage it much better than if they cannot easily make sense of what is happening to their bodies. They have a context for the sensations they are experiencing. So, Lindesmith's moment of curiosity triggered a line of scientific research that is still unfolding and bringing benefits well beyond its original application.

Key Point

These three types of problems show different aspects of the use of theory:

- To transfer the solutions of research on practical problems from one context to another.
- To develop possible solutions to a problem and to predict the likely strengths and weaknesses of alternatives.
- To connect a random question or observation to a body of established knowledge and skills that help to better understand 'what is happening here'.

CREATING THEORY

Qualitative theoretical traditions

Qualitative methods are associated with a number of different theoretical traditions in anthropology, sociology, psychology and human geography. If you go far enough back, you will also find qualitative work in economics, although this is now rare. While these traditions have their differences, our focus here is on what they have in common. Two things are important to remember.

The first is that qualitative methods are very old. In Chapter 1, we noted how you do research all the time. Of course, that has always been true. If humans had not done this, how would our species ever have colonised most of our planet? What techniques would we have used at the beginning? We would have hung out (looked and listened) and we would have asked questions and checked the answers. The core traditions of qualitative research tradition include discovery, description and verification. Counting is something that comes much later in human history, when people began keeping cattle and sheep, and modern statistical methods did not begin to appear until the 17th century. There are some newer qualitative methods: when humans developed writing, they started to create documents that recorded the ideals, values, aspirations and business of their societies in the form of individual and collective news, histories, official records and the like. From rather further back, they had also produced creative works of art, sculpture and craft that expressed ideas that were important to them, even if it is now difficult to recover what they might have meant. We have also added some new technologies: audio and video recording have allowed us to freeze and replay things that, previously, we could only hear or see once. These recordings can be shared more easily than our field notes, subject to concerns about confidentiality, such as when we observe an internet forum where people with a chronic disorder share their experiences. However, we are not really doing anything different in principle from, for example, the ancient Greek writer, Herodotus (c. 484–425BCE). He consistently distinguishes between the things he has seen for himself and those that he has learned from talking to other people. You would make exactly the same distinction: this is what people said to each other in the forum, and this is what they brought into the forum about events or feelings that others could not check for themselves. In later chapters we will look at each of these methods in detail.

Key Point

There are four main research methods in social science. The first three are qualitative and the subject of later chapters:

- *Hanging out* – watching and recording what you see and hear.
- *Asking questions* – asking people to explain what you are seeing and hearing or to tell you about things that you could not see or hear.

- *Reading the papers* – looking at the accounts that people produce for themselves, whether in official documents, personal life histories or creative arts.
- *Counting the cows* (quantitative methods) – describing people, objects, actions or events in numbers so that this information can be manipulated using mathematical techniques.

Methodology

The second thing to remember is that discussions of theory are also very old. In Chapter 1, we introduced the philosophy of knowledge or the field of *epistemology*. In this section we are going to look at a sub-field of epistemology, called *methodology*, the philosophy of method. This is the topic of some of the earliest surviving writings. How do we know what we know – and what we don't?

Zeno of Citium (c. 334BCE – c. 262BCE), who founded the Stoic school of philosophy, used to hold up his hand to illustrate the processes we are going to discuss – these were the days before PowerPoint. When we looked at our extended fingers, we were seeing something. He would then curl his fingers slightly to represent our giving attention to what we were seeing, making an observation. Then he would close his fist, representing the recognition of our observation as relevant to a theoretical scheme. Finally, he would grasp the fist with his other hand to represent the integration of that observation with the theoretical scheme as sound knowledge. (See Figures 2.1–2.4.)

These hand movements visually represent basic principles of methodology that have not changed since Zeno's time.

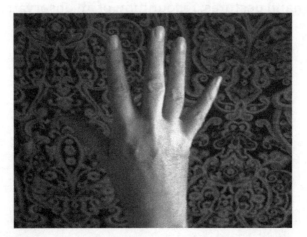

Figure 2.1 Zeno's hand gestures: seeing

Photo credit: Ed Dingwall

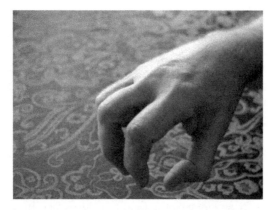

Figure 2.2   Zeno's hand gestures: making an observation

Photo credit: Ed Dingwall

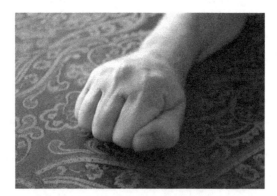

Figure 2.3   Zeno's hand gestures: recognition of an observation

Photo credit: Ed Dingwall

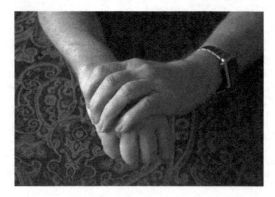

Figure 2.4   Zeno's hand gestures: integration of an observation

Photo credit: Ed Dingwall

> **Methodology** describes the process by which we come to make an observation, to decide that that our observation is sound and to integrate it with other observations to form theory, generalisable knowledge.

Definition

Zeno talked about observation, but the same principles apply to interviews, documents or artefacts: how do we come to be confident that we know what someone means by their answer to our questions in an interview or that we have correctly understood what the creator of a document, or an artefact like a painting or a statue, intended by it, explicitly or implicitly?

VIDEO SUPPORT

To put this into context, try watching M.D. Azim's video, *Research Paradigm Ontology Epistemology Methodology Methods*. You can access the video by visiting this book's online resources: https://study.sagepub.com/dingwallandstaniland.

Key Point

Try to keep these two words distinct:

- *Methodology* – the theory of method that you are using to choose tools and make sense of the data you produce with them.
- *Method* – a tool or technique for doing research.

Sometimes people like to talk about 'methodology' when they really mean 'method' because it sounds grander and more scientific. Actually, they are just being pretentious!

Induction and deduction

There are two main types of methodology, *induction* and *deduction*. (Philosophers recognise a few more, like abduction, but you need not bother with these unless you make a career in research.) These approaches are rather different, and textbooks often treat them as opposed to each other. However, most practising researchers use both, depending on which is appropriate for the problem they are investigating. The approaches are not tied to specific methods – remember the distinction between method and methodology. Although qualitative methods are often associated with induction, they can be used deductively. Similarly, some quantitative methods can be associated with inductive methodologies.

The process described by Zeno is essentially *inductive*. This kind of methodology starts from data – from observations, interviews or documents – and looks for patterns. Individual pieces of data are systematically compared with each other to identify similarities and differences. These can be given more general descriptions and assembled into logical relationships. When every piece of data is fitted into the general scheme, the scheme is accepted as valid, sound knowledge.

Induction is a good way to discover possible generalisations and to explore new situations because it involves systematic reasoning from particular items of data to a more general, theoretical, statement about what you have found. However, it is always vulnerable to what philosophers call the 'black swan' problem, as we will explain.

─────────────── FREEING OUR IMAGINATION ───────────────

For thousands of years, Europeans thought of swans as big white birds. This conclusion was based on inductive reasoning: every adult swan that a European had seen was white.

In 1697, though, a Dutch explorer called Willem de Vlamingh saw black swans in Australia. This new data showed that the 'sound knowledge' from thousands of years and countless observations in Europe was not as sound as everyone thought. The knowledge was not wrong because all the adult swans that Europeans had seen before 1697 were, indeed, white. Europeans had simply drawn the incorrect conclusion that this meant all swans everywhere were white – at least once they were fully grown. Nevertheless, until 1697, the knowledge that all adult swans are white was still useful and a practical basis for action. For example, it allowed hunters to distinguish mature and immature birds and to decide which were fit to shoot and eat.

What the black swan story tells us is that knowledge gained from induction should be treated as provisional – but it may still be better than common sense because it has been collected and analysed in a more systematic way. A good deal of clinical knowledge, for example, is assembled by inductive reasoning from the observation of particular patients. This may not be as robust as knowledge from a clinical trial but it may still improve the treatment of patients, especially where a disease or disorder is relatively uncommon or ill-defined. Researchers just need a little humility in the claims that they make for the results of induction – humility not apology because there are situations where inductive methodology is the appropriate way to proceed.

CASE STUDY SCENARIO

Induction

You stand by the hand gel dispenser at the entrance to the ward. Doctor A uses it. Doctor B uses it. Doctor C uses it ... in fact you stand there for two hours and every doctor uses it, so you conclude from your observations that 'all doctors always clean their hands'. This is inductive reasoning.

Can you see any problems with this?

The most important thing is that you have derived a general rule from a limited set of data collected in one place at one time. You cannot be sure that it will apply everywhere. Nevertheless, this may still be useful knowledge in establishing, for example, that this ward does not need to worry about doctors using the hand gel, but it might need to worry about other groups who do not use the dispenser every time.

You should also recognise that you have not yet developed a theory. You only have one case and nothing to compare it with.

You might note, too, that you are the only person who has done the observing. Have you had some effect on the doctors' behaviour? Would someone else have seen this in the same way? Are you sure you have recorded it accurately? These are problems of observer effect, reliability and validity, which we shall discuss later.

Deduction works in the opposite direction, from what is already known, or supposed, to what is unknown. You start from a theory about the world, make a prediction and try to find out whether that prediction is confirmed: if *this* is true, then *that* will happen.

Key Point

Induction – reasoning from specific cases to create general statements.
Deduction – looking for specific cases to test the truth of a general statement.

—— VIDEO SUPPORT ——

To help you understand induction and deduction, review the video *Introduction to Inductive and Deductive Reasoning*. You can access the video by visiting this book's online resources: https://study.sagepub.com/dingwallandstaniland.

In fact, for reasons like the black swan problem, it is hard to be sure that a prediction is confirmed: we cannot be sure that all doctors everywhere will pass by this hand gel dispenser. As a result, deductive research is often designed around what is called a 'null hypothesis'. This turns the prediction, or hypothesis, around so you then try to prove that it is not true. With this example, your null hypothesis might be that no doctors will use the hand gel dispenser. When you see doctors using the dispenser, you are then allowed to claim that the null hypothesis has been rejected and that its opposite must, by implication, be correct – at least in this circumstance captured by this study. Of course, this is a very simple example and we need to develop it a little further if it is going to help you when you come to do research. If we go back to the example of doctors and hand gel, a deductive approach would go something like this:

> All doctors are concerned for hand hygiene.
> There is a hand gel dispenser at the entrance to the ward.
> Prediction: All doctors will use the hand gel dispenser.
> Null hypothesis: No doctor will use the hand gel dispenser.

MOVING BETWEEN INDUCTION AND DEDUCTION – AND BACK AGAIN

We noted earlier that most practising researchers use both induction and deduction to some extent. Particular disciplines often tend to lean more in one direction than another – psychology and economics usually favour deduction, while sociology and anthropology usually favour induction. However, we think it is more useful to focus on the match between methodology and problem solving rather than getting tied up in an argument about whether one approach is better than another. As we shall often say in this book: it depends on what you are trying to achieve.

One way to explain this is to go back, yet again, to the example of the hand gel and the doctors. You have begun with an inductive phase, watching whether the doctors use the hand gel dispenser. This has allowed you to make a prediction and to test this in a deductive phase. Suppose you go to another ward and you find that only some doctors use the hand gel dispenser and others do not. You might then go back to induction and ask how the new ward differs from the one where you previously observed. What do the members of each group – gel users and non-users – have in common? What makes the two groups different from each other? This allows you to formulate a new prediction: 'only doctors who share these characteristics working on this kind of ward will use hand gel'. You can then devise tests for this prediction, looking at different groups of doctors on different wards until you have a set of statements that seem to cover every case that you can observe. This process is sometimes described as *theoretical sampling*, and we shall say more about it later. Remember, though, that this is still vulnerable to the black swan problem. Because you cannot study every case, there is always some uncertainty and you need to respect this.

Figure 2.5 may help to give you a picture of the process – you can enter and leave this at any point as long as you are clear what you are doing.

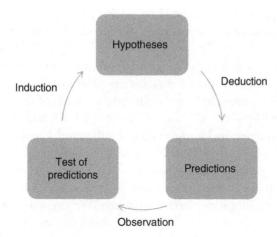

Figure 2.5   Moving between induction and deduction

Credit: Reproduced with permission from Martyn Shuttleworth (Oct 10, 2008). Hypothetico-Deductive Method. Retrieved Apr 25, 2020 from Explorable.com: https://explorable.com/hypothetico-deductive-method

There is a nice example in a classic study by Felicity Stockwell (1972) on what made patients popular and unpopular with nurses in general wards. This started as a quantitative study, but the author realised that qualitative methods were more helpful in identifying the features of the interactions between nurses and patients that led to particular judgements. In a related example, a number of medical sociologists studied the management of patients in UK accident and emergency (A&E) departments in the 1970s. Their observations led them inductively to create a theory about how the medical and nursing staff divided patients into two categories: 'good patients', who presented interesting clinical problems in areas of staff expertise; and 'bad patients', who had brought their condition on themselves, had trivial complaints, were not concerned to change their behaviour, and were unco-operative (Jeffery, 1979). However, this theory was criticised in two ways. Hughes (1980) pointed out that it did not have a good logical structure: the principles that staff were said to use to discriminate between 'good' and 'bad' patients were not opposites of each other. Hughes also observed that there were a large number of patients who were just dealt with in an entirely routine and disinterested manner. The theory could not accommodate these cases. Dingwall and Murray (1983) used Jeffery's (1979) theory to make deductive predictions about staff behaviour and showed that there was another category, 'children', who broke all the same rules as 'bad' patients but were not handled in a negative way. This led them to produce a more refined theory, where clinical features of the case and the degree to which the patient could be held responsible for their own actions both came into play to extend the classification and produce more accurate predictions of how particular patients would be treated. They also suggested, inductively, how this might vary in different locations – most of the studies had been done in teaching hospitals where there was some pressure to identify 'good' patients for learning purposes, but they had some limited data on non-teaching hospitals, which seemed to work a little differently. There might be a link, then, between the organisation of the department and the way staff classified patients and behaved towards them.

While this example shows how qualitative research can move between induction and deduction at different points, it also illustrates how theory carries ideas from one situation to another. This series of studies were done in different hospitals in different parts of the UK. All of them drew in various ways on work done by Roth (1972a, 1972b) in the USA and they have since been built on for studies in other countries, including France (Dodier and Camus, 1998; Vassy, 2001), USA (Sointu, 2017), Australia (Nugus, 2019) and Norway (Johannessen, 2019). These examples show how a series of individual case studies can build up into a bigger picture.

Theoretical development has allowed all of these different observations to be fitted into a common framework that can then inform practice anywhere. We stress the word 'inform': as we said earlier in this chapter, social science research is usually about probabilities, about ways to shift the odds in favour of doing the right thing rather than assuming that there are definitive answers for all times and all places. You might wonder whether this is enough justification, but you might think of the way in which the search for 'marginal gains' transformed British competitive cycling in the early 2000s (https://jamesclear.com/marginal-gains). This involved breaking down the system of human actions and mechanical components involved in racing a bike. By trying to improve each small part of the system by just 1 per cent, the overall performance became dramatically better. Tiny changes produced a world-beating team.

Think about this in a health care context. It is, for example, widely accepted that there are about 12,000 avoidable deaths every year in English acute hospitals. A 1 per cent improvement would save 120 lives every year, and 5×1 per cent improvements would save 600 lives. It may be more realistic to ask how we can do what we are doing just a little better than to look for one piece of magic that would improve the situation by 10 per cent.

> **Definition**
>
> Two other terms that you are likely to meet in discussions of research are validity and reliability. **Validity** refers to the accuracy of your description and **reliability** refers to the extent to which someone else collecting and analysing the same data would find the same things. Both terms are more usually associated with quantitative research methods, but they are often the basis of critical comments on qualitative research.

In quantitative research, validity is generally treated as a matter of whether a measure actually measures what it is claimed to. Does an anxiety scale, constructed by scoring the answers to a set of questions about someone's mood, measure anxiety, for example? Qualitative research is often considered to have less of a problem with validity because it is based either on data from real events or documents or from interviews that are led by the informants. In practice, though, this is not quite so straightforward. Those events still need to be recorded and then linked together as examples of more general processes. Are the records – audio, video or hand notes – accurate renderings of the original events? More importantly, how did the researcher decide which ones went together as essentially similar – and which ones were different? Did the researcher just choose nice quotes that fitted an analysis that they had already decided upon or did they allow the data to shape their conclusions?

Reliability is more troubling for qualitative research. If you have a well-designed survey questionnaire or other measurement tool, like an anxiety scale, then, in principle, it should not matter who uses it. The results should be consistent wherever and whenever the tool is applied. Qualitative research is more vulnerable to *observer effects*, where characteristics of the person and their actions influence the situation in which data are collected. When RD first studied health visitors as a young male graduate student in medical sociology, for example, his relationships to them were rather different from those that he experienced a few years later in his child protection research. By then, he had published articles from his PhD thesis in the professional magazines that health visitors read and was treated as some kind of expert who might judge practice rather than as a novice to be instructed. It became harder to ask certain questions that might seem naïve but which were important to understand how the health visitors in the later study were approaching decisions about cases. Qualitative researchers tend to deal with the problem of reliability by writing about the way in which they may have influenced the collection – and later analysis – of data. This *reflexivity* is an important feature of qualitative research reports: how did your personal characteristics like age, gender, ethnicity, sexuality and so on shape the way that people behaved when you were hanging out with them or asking them questions? We shall look at this in more detail when we come to discuss the processes of data collection.

For now, you just need to be able to recognise the potential issues of validity and reliability, and to be prepared to ask questions about them when you look at some of the materials we shall ask you to read.

A FEW WORDS ABOUT ONTOLOGY

Because this is a book about doing research, we have concentrated on introducing you to some of the basic ideas associated with epistemology, how we come to know what we think we know. However, this cannot be completely separated from another important philosophical term, *ontology*. This refers to what it is that we know. At its simplest, ontology is concerned with the question of whether there is a world 'out there' and independent of our perceptions, or whether the world is substantially, if not wholly, created by our perceptions of it.

Briefly, ideas about ontology lie along a spectrum. At one end you have the most radical forms of *constructionism* (or *constructivism* or *interpretivism*), which claim that there is nothing independent of our perceptions – or if there is, we cannot know it, because we always access it through our perceptions. We should, then, concentrate on studying our perceptions and understanding them. Various types of *phenomenology* offer methods for doing this, and have had some influence on qualitative nursing research. This is particularly evident in *autoethnography*, where the researcher focuses on understanding her own response to the situations which she encounters and what she is contributing to them (Peterson, 2015). This end of the spectrum can slide into *solipsism*, the idea that the only thing of which we can be certain is the existence of our own mind. The problems are sometimes illustrated by references to the work of George Berkeley, who was an 18th-century Irish bishop and philosopher. If the world only existed when we perceived it, what happened when we looked away? Did it stop existing? Berkeley's get-out card was to argue that the world went on existing because it was always perceived by God.

A story is told about Berkeley's contemporary, Samuel Johnson, by his biographer, James Boswell (2008 [1791]):

> After we came out of the church, we stood talking for some time together of Bishop Berkeley's ingenious sophistry to prove the nonexistence of matter, and that everything in the universe is merely ideal. I observed, that though we are satisfied his doctrine is not true, it is impossible to refute it. I never shall forget the alacrity with which Johnson answered, striking his foot with mighty force against a large stone, till he rebounded from it – 'I refute it thus'.

At the other end of the spectrum, we find the position of *objectivism* or *positivism*. This holds that there is a world of things out there which is independent of all observers. It is a single reality that is, in principle, knowable in the same way to everyone who perceives it. Most natural scientists today adopt some version of positivism as the basis of their knowledge so you will probably encounter it in other parts of your course. In many areas, this principle works quite well. However, there are some fairly obvious problems. Think of our example of miasmatic versus germ theory in the previous chapter. When we stopped explaining disease as caused by bad smells rather than by bacteria or viruses, the bad smells did not go away. We simply stopped thinking they were relevant. Think of the controversies over the explanation of mental illnesses. We may no longer explain such experiences in terms of witchcraft or demonic possession – but we cannot agree whether they result from biochemical disorders, genetic inheritance or social contexts. Consider something like a skin lesion. Is this the same object to a microbiologist who sees it as a potential environment for bacterial action, to a cellular biologist who is trying to understand the mechanisms of growth and repair, to a surgeon who is considering whether some intervention might be necessary, or to a nurse who needs to select the right kind of dressing?

Although you will find qualitative researchers who take most positions along this spectrum, with the possible exception of the hardest forms of positivism, they tend to cluster around an intermediate position known as *realism*. This accepts the idea of an independent, external reality. There is a world out there, made up of material objects that constrain human possibilities for action. You cannot run 100 metres with a broken leg. If you are flying an aeroplane, you cannot treat a mountain range as a social construct. At the same time, we can only know this world through our perceptions of it, which leaves room for uncertainty, disagreement and interpretation. Those perceptions are also constrained by the language that we used to communicate them. We have to translate our perceptions into words or images in order to share them. As we do so, we transform them from purely private observations into a way of looking at the world that we have in common with other people. This is what social scientists usually mean when they talk about 'culture' – the shared values, beliefs and knowledge of some group as expressed through their language, art, stories and other symbols. Culture shapes how we learn about the world and how we communicate our experiences. The German sister in the previous chapter was articulating a different nursing culture from that which we might teach or learn today, but which reflected her past training. At the same time, the world pushes back – her ward was full of hazards that were not recognised by the culture of practice that had shaped her professional development.

This is a complicated area of philosophy and we have drastically simplified it here. If you want to know more about these issues, you should go on to a more specialised introduction like Hollis (2002) or Williams (2016).

CHAPTER SUMMARY POINTS

In this chapter we have introduced you to some different research problem types and we are sure you will be able to think of many more. We have discussed some of the challenges in defining practical, theoretical and curiosity problems and introduced you to some important terminologies involved with qualitative research. Try at this stage to remember the differences between inductive and deductive reasoning as you will need this later to help you decide on your own best research approach in order to answer prospective research questions which we will be covering in the next chapter.

FURTHER READING

The literature in this area can get technical very quickly. However, there are two relatively short books, by Howard Becker, that we would recommend. Becker is one of the most important and influential sociologists of the last half century. These books are his attempt to set down, in an accessible form, the lessons that he has passed on to his own students for nearly seventy years.

Becker, H.S. (1998) *Tricks of the Trade: How to think about your research while you're doing it.* Chicago, IL: University of Chicago Press.

Becker, H.S. (2017) *Evidence.* Chicago, IL: University of Chicago Press.

Another useful, and perhaps more immediately practical, book is:

Booth, W.C., Colomb, G.C., Williams, J.M., Bizup, H. and Fitzgerald, W.T. (2016) *The Craft of Research* (4th edn). Chicago, IL: University of Chicago Press.

If you would like to know more about the Stoics, this is an accessible introduction:

Sellars, J. (2019) *Lessons in Stoicism: What ancient philosophers teach us about how to live.* London: Allen Lane.

3

Creating a Project

Learning Outcomes

At the end of this chapter you will be able to:

- Identify the differences between research topics, research problems, and research purposes
- Create problem statements, research strategies and research questions

In the last chapter, we introduced you to some different types of research problem. We discussed the challenges in defining practical, theoretical and curiosity problems and described some important terminologies associated with qualitative research. Parts of that chapter had to be quite abstract because you need to understand why theory and methodology are important for health care researchers. This chapter, though, is more practical. It will consolidate the material we have introduced in the previous chapters by working through another example of how to turn a practice issue into a research problem. Along the way, we will look at the process of defining researchable questions and deciding how to investigate them.

We have already introduced the different ways in which research projects can originate – from simple curiosity to finding a solution to a practice problem. We have suggested how you could start to think about moving from a problem to a project and we have taken you through some of the ways in which you might study something like the use of hand gel. We are now going to revisit some of these topics by working through an example from something that is common to almost all clinical nursing work – oral care. This will put more emphasis on practice than curiosity as a source of research problems, which is often the case in nursing. However, you should not forget how important curiosity can be: just asking 'Why are we doing this?' or 'Why is this happening' has led to key discoveries and innovations in many fields.

TERMINOLOGY

Before we work through our case study, let us reintroduce some terms that you may have already met and define them more formally.

- *Research topic* – the broadest description of the subject to be investigated.
- *Research problem* – the aspect or element of the topic that is going to be the focus of attention in a research project.
- *Research purpose* – what the project is intended to achieve: its intention or objective.
- *Research question* – the translation of the research problem into one (or more) specific questions to be investigated by a research project.

Research topic

In health care research, research topics are often related to particular clinical areas. If you are working in a surgical area, for example, 'post-operative care' could be an example of a research topic. This is a very general and high-level description of where some research might be directed. Issues like 'care of the elderly', 'childbirth' or 'patient safety' are at the same level. You cannot investigate a research topic directly (it is too vague) but it signals the beginning of the process of concentrating attention that is the first step in all research projects. You are going to look *here* rather than *there*.

─────────────────── **VIDEO SUPPORT** ───────────────────

The video *How to Develop a Good Research Topic* will help you with the development of a research topic. You can access the video by visiting this book's online resources: https://study.sagepub.com/dingwallandstaniland.

Research problem

Having identified a research topic, the next step is to identify part of it that makes a more manageable research problem: *progressive focusing* is an important aspect of all qualitative research. If 'post-operative care' is your research topic, 'post-operative care for people who have had bariatric surgery' might be a research problem. For example, are the ways in which nursing care has traditionally been provided after surgery equally appropriate for obese patients who have received gastric bands? In qualitative research, you may sometimes not need to go any further, especially when the work is exploratory: trying to find out what is happening and how more specific studies should be designed. A research problem may also direct a programme of work where different projects focus on particular questions but all contribute to a broader understanding of the issue. More commonly, though, especially with student dissertations, you need to take two more steps.

——————————————— **VIDEO SUPPORT** ———————————————

The video *Identifying a Research Problem* will help you with the development of a research problem. You can access the video by visiting this book's online resources: https://study.sagepub.com/dingwallandstaniland.

_____

Research purpose

This step asks you to think about what you hope to achieve by your research. Are you actually asking a scientific question? For example, you will often find people with a strong commitment to a particular policy, technique or intervention saying that they want to do research to 'prove' that it works (or that the alternatives do not)? If you think about this statement, you might wonder whether what they are doing should be called research and, indeed, whether there is any point in it. If you already know the outcome you want, can we trust you to do the research impartially and to be ready to accept that it might produce the 'wrong' answer? Are you just pretending to do research, using qualitative or quantitative methods to put on a show that might persuade people to agree with you? As you read more qualitative studies, you will find this quite often happens. The authors pick nice quotations from interviews or tell stories from their fieldwork that fit the conclusion they always wanted to reach.

A related point is the need to recognise when you are asking questions that are really moral or ethical rather than factual. Research often informs moral and ethical debates, but it cannot replace them. Questions like 'Should women be able to access abortion on demand?' or 'Should euthanasia be legalised' are not in themselves researchable. Research may tell us whether women's experience of abortion is positive or negative and what contributes to that assessment. However, it does not give us answers to questions about the relative weight we should give to concerns for individual liberty and human dignity. We might, hypothetically, show that experiences of abortion are overwhelmingly negative but still prefer a commitment to the individual's liberty to take that risk rather than a paternalist restriction on access. Arguments about liberty, paternalism and human dignity draw on other sources in moral philosophy, ethics and political theory. You may need to know about them, but you should not confuse them with the design and practice of research.

——————————————— **VIDEO SUPPORT** ———————————————

Purpose Part 1: General guidance for writing the research purpose for qualitative and qualitative and Purpose Part 2: Qualitative purpose wording for writing a research proposal, publication or thesis may be helpful videos at this stage. You can access the videos by visiting this book's online resources: https://study.sagepub.com/dingwallandstaniland.

_____

Research question

Finally, we end up with the research question. In quantitative research, these are often written in formal ways as hypotheses to be tested. Some qualitative researchers tend to be less formal, but if you try to define your research by one question, you can check whether you are starting off from the right place. Does the question imply that you already know the answer? Is this really a question about values rather than facts? *Your question will also help you to check whether you should be using qualitative methods at all.* They are best suited to answering questions about what is going on rather than questions about how often something is happening. There are, for example, many comparative studies of death rates – how many people died in a particular hospital, locality or country from a particular cause in a given time period. You would not use qualitative methods to analyse these differences. However, those rates are produced by decisions about what is written on death certificates and how it is coded – we shall say more about this in Chapter 8. There are many studies that show great variation in these practices, with obvious implications for the conclusions that are drawn from quantitative studies. If you work in a cancer treatment service, you may want to benchmark your performance by comparing your outcomes with those of other similar services, adjusted for various risk factors. If you want to know how those outcomes are produced, you need to look at what is happening within the services.

VIDEO SUPPORT

Watch *Qualitative research questions: Where, why and how questions are used in research proposals* to bring this all together. You can access the video by visiting this book's online resources: https://study.sagepub.com/dingwallandstaniland.

FREEING OUR IMAGINATION

Framing a researchable question

Developing an overarching question is useful at the start of a qualitative study to capture the basic goal, but there needs to be a clarity which will help the reader to gain a picture of what the research is about. This also comes with practice and gains focus as the study progresses.

For example:

What is the experience of living with diabetes?

The question here is very broad and not really clear; we don't know whether the study will look at people with insulin dependent diabetes or non-insulin dependent diabetes, or at people who are living with a diabetic person. A second attempt of this overarching question could be:

What is it like to be an insulin dependent diabetic?

Ultimately a clear picture may emerge to encapsulate the study:

How do you live with diabetes? Exploring the lives of insulin dependent diabetics.

The questions are open but manage to direct some focus for a literature review and the inquiry process.
Another question might be:

Why do people self-harm?

This again is broad, and it will be extremely difficult to provide a full explanation by undertaking a qualitative research study. The focus could be improved to:

What explanations do teenagers give for self-harm?

Ultimately this could be incorporated into a study title:

An exploration of self-harm in teenagers: what explanations do teenagers give for self-harm?

This is clearer and appears more interesting. It is still flexible and can be modified depending on the findings from a literature review.
Other examples of qualitative questions for nursing might include:

- What happens when patients get transferred from one ward to another? Is any information lost?
- How do the members of a multidisciplinary team understand their role in ensuring the safe delivery of care?

Try to develop these questions further to give a better picture as to what the studies might be about.

Where do research questions come from? There are two main sources. The first is from your own experience. You may remember, from Chapter 1, that we encouraged you to be ready to ask questions about why things happened in a particular way in the place where you were working or studying. It was not acceptable to answer 'Because that's how we do it here' or 'Because we have always done it this way'. KS experienced this as a patient, when she told a nurse that she was worried that a newly-applied plaster edge was already digging into the line of sutures over a fresh surgical wound. The response was 'I "always" do the dressings this way'; this nurse was 'always' causing discomfort to patients, discounting the patient's actual experience, and not offering a rationale for her technique. (In this case the dressing had to be re-applied two days later because of increasing discomfort and swelling.)

If you are trying to find the evidence to inform your practice, you would start by looking for very specific literature investigating this question – we shall describe this process in the next chapter. If you cannot find any specific studies, you would then move up a level (research problem) to see whether research had been done in similar areas that might guide you – perhaps you have a problem with skin care in people with dementia. You cannot find any research directly about this, but you can find reports about research on skin care for people with advanced diabetes. This knowledge might transfer, or it might offer models that you could adapt for research with your group of patients. Suppose, just for the sake of argument, you did not find anything about skin care with any patient group relevant to your concerns. You could then move up another level (research topic) to ask what research has been done about the factors that contribute to maintaining, or disrupting, the integrity of human skin. You could then move back down to the challenge of developing evidence-based practice for the patients you are actually working with.

The second source of research questions is from your own reading. Chapter 2 contained several examples of where ideas moved between very different research sites in ways that helped to understand each of them. One of these could be 'emotional labour', where research on nursing has borrowed an idea from a study of women flight attendants (Hochschild, 1983). Experienced qualitative researchers usually read quite widely outside their own immediate field, looking for this sort of transfer. Nursing has traditionally been more focused on its own concerns and it obviously takes time to build a wider stock of knowledge from reading. Nevertheless, there is a lot to be learned from reading studies of how other professions interact with their clients or service users, how different kinds of organisations function, how gender affects careers and opportunities in other occupations and so on. Even reading about research on nursing in other countries can help to prompt you to ask 'Does this happen here too – and if not, why not?' The same hierarchy works here too. There is, for example, a literature about how to break 'bad news', which both looks upwards to very general research on how people talk to each other and downwards to the various occupations and work sites where bad news may be broken. One of the nice things about qualitative research reports is that they are often inherently interesting or tell you about corners of the world you would be unlikely ever to encounter.

To explain this, we use an example which is outside the health care field, but which could help us to understand some reasons why staff in nursing homes, for example, might exploit patients. Staci Newmahr (2011) carried out a participant observation study of a private club for sadomasochists as the basis of her PhD. She discovered that this group had a strong ethic of mutual care. There were collective understandings about the boundaries of acceptable behaviour and the responsibilities of 'tops' towards 'bottoms'. People who did not respect these boundaries or their responsibilities would be excluded from the community. You might also want to think about the scandals around sexual harassment in entertainment, sport and politics, which were accepted as 'normal' and went unnoticed for many years. People around the star performers who perpetrated the abuse just cleaned up afterwards without thinking about their moral collusion in the behaviour (Chen et al., 2019).

What might this have to say to nursing? Well, you could think about the way in which several scandals have revealed nurses treating patients in ways that are considered to be cruel or abusive. Critics often explain this as an individual failure, a lack of compassion by the nurses involved. They call for more psychological tests or training in empathy. Newmahr's work suggests that these abuses might stem from the way in which any social group comes to set and maintain standards of behaviour for its members. You could compare it, for example, with Stannard's (1973) study of patient abuse in a small US nursing home. Newmahr's sado-masochists had a strongly-shared culture and were highly visible to each other. The culture in Stannard's nursing home was weakly shared between nurses and aides, whose actions were largely invisible to each other. If the culture and structure of the group are the source of problems with the standard of care, then a focus on individual behaviour may not be an effective solution. The challenge is to change the collective benchmark, and the means by which members of the group maintain it, rather than the individuals applying it.

Let us try to pull some of this together with the example of a project on oral care.

CASE STUDY SCENARIO

Suppose your regular job is nursing on a high dependency unit. You have been off duty over a weekend. When you return to work, you notice that some patients' mouths appear to be 'dirty'. The staff going off duty assure you that they have carried out oral care as required by local policy and practice.

- Is 'oral care' a research topic, a research problem or a research question?

  'Oral care' is a research topic – a very general description of an area for investigation.

- Do you now have a *research problem*?

  Yes. Your attention is now focused on 'oral care in high dependency patients'.

- What contributes to this?

  You need to find out.

(Continued)

(Continued)

- Do you have a research purpose?

  Yes. As a conscientious professional, you do not think that it is acceptable for patients to have 'dirty' mouths, which may cause distress and potentially other health problems.

- Do you have a research question?

  No. You still need to work out what, specifically, you are going to do to find out why these 'dirty' mouths are occurring. You also need to decide whether this is a qualitative or a quantitative research question. Are you asking how many patients have poor oral care or how come patients happen to have poor oral care? The first question can only be answered by quantitative methods; the second question is most likely to be best answered by qualitative methods.

How are you going to work out what your research question is? A distinctive feature of the social science traditions that created qualitative research methods is the way they insist on *analysing* the possible research questions before they start. This is not always a comfortable thing to do. In this case, for example, the hospital management might think the question is:

'Why don't nurses on this unit follow our policies properly?'

However, this has ruled out an important alternative question:

'Does this hospital have the right policies to secure oral care on units like this one?'

Remember our discussion of Lindesmith's (1965) work in the previous chapter and the way in which it led social scientists to ask whether the harm caused to addicts by their illegal drug use resulted from the drugs or from the laws that defined them as criminals. Turning the question round in this way has not made social scientists very popular – and asking whether your managers have got their policy right may not make you very popular! However, it is what a scientific approach requires.

Where do you start, then? Remember that we said there were three basic methods of qualitative research: hanging out, asking questions, and reading the papers. When you are working in an area that is rich in documents, this will always be the place to start. In a research project, you will find three kinds of documents; remember that documents are not just material on paper but also pictures, websites, social media pages or posts, video or other recordings, and material objects like nursing uniforms or the statues that stand in the hospital's entrance. The three types of document are:

- The documents produced by an organisation – in this case a hospital – to record and govern its own activity. Oral care may be the subject of a written protocol, entries in patient records, and regular management reports that summarise the record entries. The hospital may also produce documents for outside audiences to promote a favourable image of its work and attract patients or to satisfy auditors from the bodies that check whether it is spending money properly or delivering good quality care.
- The documents produced about an organisation, reviewing and commenting on its activity. These include the assessment and feedback reports from auditors and quality reviewers. This category would also cover the local and national media coverage: press, TV, radio, social media, patient feedback websites. What do these sources have to say about this hospital, or about other hospitals that are rather like it?
- The research literature published in scientific journals, monographs or the 'grey' zone of commissioned reports. We shall look at these more closely in the next chapter on literature reviews.

In our oral care project, though, we would be trying to understand what was already known about the problem:

- How does the hospital govern and document oral care? Is there a policy statement, guideline, or protocol? If so, when and how was this created? How is the policy translated to the people who actually deliver the care? Is it on a noticeboard or an intranet site? Are there regular training events to communicate it? Is the administration of oral care recorded on patient notes? If so, are the entries checked and countersigned? Are there regular statistical reports to managers summarising these records?
- Are you the only person who is worried about the standard of oral care in this hospital? Have quality reviewers, patients or relatives already been complaining? If no one else has noticed, are you being too picky or are you seeing something at an early stage that will eventually become a serious issue?
- What else do we know about oral care? What does microbiological, dental and nursing practice research identify as the risks and challenges – and the interventions that might help to manage these?

Once you have assembled this information, you are in a better place to decide what your research question should be and what methods to use to answer it. Suppose, for example, you find that the hospital protocol for oral care was written ten years ago, can only be read in an obscure location on an intranet site that most nurses cannot easily access, and is not picked up in patient records or management reports. This would suggest that your research question might be something like 'How come this hospital works in this way?'; on the other hand, perhaps the protocol was recently reviewed and modified in the light of current research and actively publicised through internal refresher training events. Your question might then be something like 'How come the nurses on this unit do not comply with the protocol?'

At this point, it is a good idea to write a problem statement. Whatever the length of your dissertation, this will serve as an early draft of the opening sections, or chapters, on the background and context of the research and on the literature review. The problem statement preserves the history of your own thinking – how you came to do this particular study in this particular way. It also provides a useful way to test your thinking with your supervisor, advisor or dissertation committee.

You should create a folder to hold all of your drafts – we shall suggest writing other working documents in later chapters. When you come to write the final version of your report, dissertation or thesis, you will draw on these documents. This is exactly how we wrote this book. The folder might be virtual on your computer, or it might be physical. Some of our students still find it useful to have a cardboard or plastic file for each chapter of their assignment, where they can put hard copies of drafts, relevant materials or working notes. When they come to write the final text, they spread it all out on a table, desk or floor and organise it from there. Other students are happy to do this electronically, with a sub-folder for the drafts of each chapter and a parallel sub-folder of resources, for PDF copies of papers or notes that they have made as ideas came to them. Find out which works best for you, but always remember to have a backup copy as well. Do not throw anything away until the project is complete and your course's assessment processes are finished.

CRITICAL THINKING EXERCISE

Writing a problem statement

You can use either our example or one of your own. The statement should contain the following components:

Research topic

- What is this research about? This should be very brief and general. It is a version of the 'elevator pitch'. This gets its name from Hollywood folklore that a film promoter may only get the length of an elevator journey – allegedly 11 seconds - to catch the attention of a potential backer. In the same way, this should be a non-technical description of your project in no more than a couple of sentences. You should keep coming back to this and polishing it as your study progresses. In our case study, it might be something like: 'This is a study of oral care and why patients who need it don't get it.'

Research problem

- What would be an ideal state of affairs?
  - Who says so?
  - On what evidence?
  - How good is the evidence?
  - Do they have any particular reason for making this claim - getting more resources, status, privilege and so on?
- What actually seems to be happening?
  - Who says so?
  - On what evidence?
  - How good is the evidence?
  - Do they have any particular reason for making this claim - getting more resources, status, privilege and so on?

Research purpose

- Does it matter if the ideal and the reality do not match?
  - What are the consequences?
  - Is the imperfection big enough to justify spending time and resources on a research project?
  - Are the ideals set too high?
  - Are the ideals reflecting altruism, self-interest or, most commonly, some mix of both?
- Why should we care if reality falls short?

Research question

- What do I need to know to understand how come things come to happen this way?
  - In this example, how patients come to receive the oral care that they get.

THE RESEARCH STRATEGY

The problem statement justifies your decision to look at a particular question. It is important to recognise that in qualitative research, that question may well continue to evolve as the study progresses. When you have an opportunity to look more closely at a research site, you may find things that you missed in your original review. There is nothing wrong with this and it is one of the real strengths of qualitative research. However, it is also important that you assemble as good a picture as you can before you start so that you can develop an efficient and effective strategy for your fieldwork.

Some writers about qualitative methods suggest that you should just go into a site and hang around to see what happens. If there really is no other relevant work and you have ample time and resources, this is what could be done. However, that advice often reflects the situation of fifty or sixty years ago, when there was much less research literature and experience with the systematic use of qualitative methods in the social sciences. Today, we can use that body of work to anticipate where it is most likely to be productive to focus our efforts, at least at the beginning of our investigations. One of the pioneers of qualitative research, the anthropologist Bronisław Malinowski, wrote that if someone

> sets out on an expedition, determined to prove certain hypotheses, … is incapable of changing [their] views constantly and casting them off ungrudgingly under the pressure of evidence, needless to say [the] work will be worthless … Preconceived ideas are pernicious in any scientific work, but *foreshadowed problems* are the main endowment of a scientific thinker. (1922: 9, emphasis added),

Let us come back to the two questions that we identified from the oral care example: is the poor oral care the result of a problem with the protocol for delivery or with the nurses who are supposed to be implementing it? These foreshadow problems in different ways, with quite different implications for the design and direction of the project.

———————— FREEING OUR IMAGINATION ————————

Before you read any further, make some notes about how you would investigate each of these possible questions:

- Why is the oral care protocol not having any impact on nursing practice?
- Why are nurses not implementing the oral care protocol?

Keep these notes and compare them with the following approaches we suggest.

The protocol is the problem

Suppose your document review finds that the oral care protocol was written a long time ago, is hidden in an obscure place and is never drawn to anyone's attention. You might think that this is a scandal. That may well be true, but it is not actually a helpful response. Once upon a time, someone, or some group of people, obviously spent time creating the document, deciding where to place it, and planning what to do with it. In a busy organisation like a hospital, they would not just do this for their own amusement. Your project, then, would be to write a history of this process. You might look for more documents from the drafting process and go and talk to people who were involved in that (we shall tell you more about these methods in later chapters). You might ask why the organisation set about writing the protocol – was this a requirement of some outside agency? You might ask what was done with the protocol at the time – was it heavily promoted on one occasion to staff or was it just shown to the agency that had asked for it as evidence that the work had been done? You might look at the processes by which similar protocols are still being written and revised – you could observe these, which would give you better data than relying on people's memories of what happened a few years ago. This was a core element of KS's own PhD thesis (Staniland, 2007), where she observed a quality assurance process in a major hospital and showed that it made little impact on the quality of patient care, but pleased external audiences. It still had a positive benefit to the hospital, though, because it received more money and won awards that enhanced its reputation.

This kind of lateral thinking can be very powerful. Increasingly, social scientists are starting from a material object, like a policy document, as a focus for studying the work that goes on around it. One of RD's PhD students, Rachel Hale (2016), investigated the uptake of influenza vaccination by staff in some Welsh hospitals. This has often been framed as a question about why health care workers don't get vaccinated, leading to disciplinary threats from hospital employers and professional bodies for non-compliance. Rachel asked how the vaccine travelled from the factory to the injection site in the health care worker's arm. She showed that this journey had all kinds of obstacles at every stage. Resistance by health care workers was a fairly minor part of the explanation for limited uptake. It was really not fair to blame them until the other barriers had been reduced or eliminated. Telling the story from the vaccine's point of view made it look quite different. In the same way, you could think about how you would tell the story of oral care in this hospital from the protocol's point of view. How would it travel from the committee that wrote it to the nurses who were supposed to implement it? What competition would it face along the way from other hospital priorities?

The nurses are the problem

The other possibility that we identified was that the problem with oral care resulted from the nurses on the unit. The protocol was up to date, well publicised, and regularly promoted through induction and in-service training. However, your observations of 'dirty' mouths showed that the nurses simply did not follow it. Your starting point here will almost certainly be observational, if possible – we shall explain later why this is generally considered to be the *gold standard* for qualitative research.

The question in this respect would be 'What is happening on this unit that means the nurses are not providing adequate oral care?' Again, it is important not to rush to judgement and assume that you are dealing with a group of people who are sloppy and uncaring. They may be, but then you have to ask how it is possible for such practice to arise and go unchecked, as we noted earlier in comparing the work of Newmahr and Stannard. 'Hanging out' should enable you to see what the nurses are actually doing and help you to generate further questions:

- Where does oral care fit within the set of tasks that they are expected to perform within a shift?
- What priority does it receive when they are busy?
- What is their understanding about the role of a protocol? (Contemporary nursing puts a lot of emphasis on the importance of independent professional judgement, so the nurses may treat the protocol as optional.)

- Does the unit have a lot of casually employed nurses who are not exposed to the hospital's publicity and training?
- Do supervisors pick up on oral care when they are monitoring the nurses' work?
- Do visitors notice and draw it to the attention of staff?

You might now want to supplement the observation with interviews – or, if time and resources are short, you might have to do the whole project by means of interviews.

RESEARCH DESIGN OR RESEARCH STRATEGY?

It is now time to go back to your problem statement and to extend this with a plan that sets out what you are going to do. Quantitative researchers would usually call this a 'research design', but qualitative researchers tend to think of it as a research strategy. A research design would be quite precise – we are going to survey 250 people from this patient group by taking every fifth name from this set of clinical records or we are going to survey the general population by recruiting 1,000 people and setting our interviewers' quotas to ensure that the sample includes the right proportions by gender, economic status, ethnicity and so on.

A research strategy extends the idea of foreshadowing but leaves some flexibility. In our first example, you could state your intention to talk to everyone involved in drafting the original protocol, which would give you an estimate of the number of interviews. However, you might find that it is also important to talk to other people, say the chief executive or the person in their office who decided to set up a drafting committee or someone from the training side who might have been responsible for telling nurses about the document. In our second example, you might think about how long you would need to observe practice on the unit to see enough oral care to find out what was thought to be routine and acceptable. This would certainly need to include observations at different times of day and different days of the week. We shall say more later about how to make these sorts of sampling decisions. For the moment, your strategy might just describe the factors that you think would be relevant.

Keep your problem statement handy because you should come back to it from time to time as we go through the next two chapters. These will explain in more detail how to carry out a literature and background review and how to turn your problem statement into a research proposal. As we said, you will also need it when you come to write the final text of your assignment.

───────────────────────── **VIDEO SUPPORT** ─────────────────────────

To help put this all together it may be helpful to watch *How to Write a Central Question for a Qualitative Research Study, Thesis, Publication and Proposal*. You can access the video by visiting this book's online resources: https://study.sagepub.com/dingwallandstaniland.

CHAPTER SUMMARY POINTS

In this chapter we have moved on from the more abstract discussions of the first two chapters to apply their approach in practice. We have discussed how to identify research topics, research problems and research purposes in order to create problem statements, research strategies and research questions. This is the beginning of writing a good proposal for your project or dissertation. The next step will be to review current, relevant, literature, which we turn to in the next chapter.

FURTHER READING

A good deal of qualitative research relevant to nursing is published in the following journals. This is quite a long list, but you should not feel compelled to read each one so much as to know that it exists and roughly what sorts of material you might find there.

Qualitative Health Research (*QHR*) is a peer-reviewed monthly journal that provides an international, interdisciplinary forum to enhance health care and further the development and understanding of qualitative research in health care settings.

Merner, B., Hill, S., and Taylor, M. (2019) '"I'm trying to stop things before they happen": Carers' contributions to patient safety in hospitals', *Qualitative Health Research*, 29(10): 1508–518. Available at https://doi.org/10.1177/1049732319841021 (accessed 25/2/20).

Viergever, R.F. (2019) 'The critical incident technique: method or methodology?', *Qualitative Health Research*, 29(7): 1065–79. Available at https://doi.org/10.1177/1049732318813112 (accessed 25/2/20).

Qualitative Research in Medicine and Healthcare provides readers with peer-reviewed articles that examine: the illness experience from multiple and varied perspectives; constructions of health, illness and health care that highlight relational and global contexts; health care policies in various organisational and institutional settings; the pressures of neoliberalism on health care; attention to the communicative dynamics of the patient–provider relationship; narrative approaches to health.

Britt, R. and Englebert, A. (2019) 'Experiences of patients living with inflammatory bowel disease in rural communities', *Qualitative Research in Medicine and Healthcare*, 3(1): 40–46. Available at https://doi.org/10.4081/qrmh.2019.7962 (accessed 25/2/20).

Meluch, A. (2018) 'Above and beyond: an exploratory study of breast cancer patient accounts of healthcare provider information-giving practices and informational support', *Qualitative Research in Medicine and Healthcare*, 2(2): 113–20. Available at https://doi.org/10.4081/qrmh.2018.7387 (accessed 25/2/20).

International Journal of Qualitative Studies on Health and Well-being (QHW) is an Open Access peer-reviewed scientific journal that acknowledges the international and interdisciplinary nature of health-related issues.

Magnussen, I-L., Alteren, J. and Bondas, T. (2019) 'Appreciative inquiry in a Norwegian nursing home: a unifying and maturing process to forward new knowledge and new practice', *International Journal of Qualitative Studies on Health and Well-being*, 14(1). Available at www.tandfonline.com/doi/full/10.1080/17482631.2018.1559437 (accessed 24/2/20).

Finally, remember to extend your search for an article beyond your subject area:

Kim, E-K., Park, E.Y., Gong, J-W.S., Jang, S-H., Choi, Y-H. and Lee, H-K. (2017) 'Lasting effect of an oral hygiene care program for patients with stroke during in-hospital rehabilitation: a randomized single-center clinical trial', *Disability and Rehabilitation*, 39(22): 2324–9. Available at https://doi.org/10.1080/09638288.2016.1226970 (accessed 24/2/20).

Preus, H.R., Maharajasingam, N., Rosic, J. and Baelum, V. (2019) 'Oral hygiene phase revisited: how different study designs have affected results in intervention studies', *Journal of Clinical Periodontology*, 46(5): 548–51. Available at https://doi.org/10.1111/jcpe.13109 (accessed 24/2/20).

You should also be aware of these journals, which publish some nursing content:

Sociology of Health & Illness is an international journal that publishes sociological articles on all aspects of health, illness, medicine and health care. This is particularly useful for finding more theoretically-informed work that draws on a wider range of influences.

Social Science and Medicine provides an international and interdisciplinary forum for the dissemination of social science research on health. This is helpful for its international reach and tends to include more applied research, especially from developing countries.

We have also encouraged you to think about how to read more widely and to see what other topics are being examined by qualitative researchers. You need not read these two journals cover to cover, just look at the contents pages or abstracts to get a feel for what is out there:

Journal of Contemporary Ethnography is an international and interdisciplinary forum for research using ethnographic methods to examine human behaviour in natural settings.

Symbolic Interaction is a quarterly peer-reviewed academic journal and covers research and theoretical developments concerned with symbolic interactionism, which is one of the major sociological traditions in qualitative research.

Two books that you might find useful are:

Loseke, D. (2016) *Methodological Thinking: Basic Principles of Social Research Design* (2nd edn). Thousand Oaks, CA: Sage.

Loseke, D. (2017) *Thinking about Social Problems: An Introduction to Constructionist Perspectives*. New York: Routledge.

4

Reviewing the Literature

Learning Outcomes

At the end of this chapter you will be able to:

- Identify relevant literature
- Define a literature review
- Explain a search strategy
- Search relevant literature systematically
- Read and analyse the literature relevant to the problem
- Make sense of the literature
- Critically read and judge the quality of qualitative research articles
- Organise the results
- Report findings from the literature
- Read and review research reports, journal articles, book chapters or books

This chapter will discuss reviewing the literature. It goes into quite a lot of detail, but, depending on your level of experience, you can use it either as a step-by-step guide or as revision for points you may have forgotten.

The activities in the first three chapters of this book have helped you to develop your ideas about what a research topic might be and how you might approach it. However, you still need to define how this is going to build on what other people have previously done (or not done), and to see what you can learn from their experiences.

Imagine all the studies that have previously been written as bricks in a wall of knowledge. This is the fourth action described by Zeno of Citium, who you met in Chapter 2, where his hands clasped each other to symbolise that an observation is secure and integrated with other observations. In the same way, the strength of a wall comes from the bonds between the bricks and the ways in which they overlap and embrace each other. Your project, however small-scale, will add another brick to the wall.

First, you need to decide where that brick is likely to go. Are you trying to fill a hole? Are you trying to check whether another brick is correctly placed? Are you trying to add extra substance, to build a buttress and give more strength to the wall by putting your study directly alongside another one? More rarely, you might even find that nobody has ever tried to build a wall in this particular spot, and it will be your job to lay out the foundation. This is the work of a literature review.

Before you start a new project, you need to describe what is already known – and not known – in order to show what your study is intended to add. Of course, the extent to which you do this will depend on the time and resources available. An undergraduate or master's level dissertation will not be able to dig as deeply as a PhD thesis or a project that is designed specifically to bring together everything that has been written about a topic, either to decide on best practice or to define where there are gaps that need further research. The principles, though, are the same at any scale.

This chapter will explain how to do a literature review in a 'systematic fashion' so you can assure your readers that there is unlikely to be any significant work that you have overlooked. It is important to note, though, that this is not quite the same as doing a 'systematic review', which is a special kind of literature review that we will describe later.

You should also remember the point that we have been emphasising in previous chapters, namely the importance of wider reading. Papers in professional journals are often structured in ways that make them easy to search in terms of problems that have already been recognised. Wider reading is a way to find new ideas that help you to look at professional practice in different ways that might suggest novel solutions to problems – or identify emerging problems that have not yet been recognised by the profession.

When you have worked through this chapter, you should be able to arrange your literature review around a basic structure such as:

- Defining a search strategy
- Searching systematically
- Appraising the evidence
- Organising the results

WHAT IS A LITERATURE REVIEW?

You may be asked to write a literature review as a separate assignment; more often, it will form part of the introduction to an essay, research report, or thesis. The main purpose of a literature review is to tell readers about the established knowledge and ideas on a topic, and to identify their strengths and weaknesses.

A literature review describes and analyses what has been published on a topic by recognised scholars and researchers.

A **narrative** or traditional **literature review** is a comprehensive, critical and objective analysis of the current knowledge on a topic. Such a review is an essential part of the research process and helps to establish a theoretical framework and focus or context for your research. (This is the most usual approach in social science research.)

A **systematic literature review** is a type of literature review that uses a systematic described method to collect secondary data, critically appraise research studies, and synthesise findings qualitatively or quantitatively. It is designed to provide a complete, exhaustive summary of current evidence relevant to a research question.

Definition

Key Point

In a research study, the scope of the literature review is defined by a guiding concept (e.g. your research objective, the problem or issue you are discussing or the argument of your thesis). A review is not just a descriptive list of the material available, but an interpretive, thoughtful analysis which helps to *build a case* about why your study is important and *how* it will fill a gap in the literature.

A literature review tells you what research has already been completed on a given subject. By finding out what is already known, you can identify neglected or unexplored areas – 'gaps in the literature' – into which your own project can be fitted. You can also learn from the practical experiences of other researchers, especially about their choice of methods and how well that worked for them. This information will help you to understand what approaches have succeeded (and failed) so you can benefit in designing and carrying out your own research project.

You may find that nobody has previously written much on the subject that you are interested in. You should not be discouraged by this. As we have already suggested, you can ask what other cases might be similar – or different – and see what has been written about them. If you still do not find very much material, then you just have a stronger argument for doing the research. The important thing is to show that you have looked, which means keeping a good record of your searches.

VIDEO SUPPORT

It may help you at this stage to watch *How to Write a Literature Review in 30 Minutes or Less*. You can access the video by visiting this book's online resources: https://study.sagepub.com/dingwallandstaniland, or the text version is available at http://polaris.umuc.edu/ewc/lit_review/Step5.html (accessed 26/2/20).

If you are studying for a qualification, you should have access to a professional library. Make friends with the library staff. They will run courses that show you how to use the specific search tools and databases that are available in their library. However, they also have a lot of good advice to offer about how and where to look for material, and how to keep track of what you have been doing. Make sure that you know how to access the library from home as it is entirely possible to conduct a good literature review online without spending hours in the library.

Key Point

This is a moment to identify two important lessons:

- Keep a detailed record of how you search for material, especially your decisions about what to include and exclude.
- Make sure you log the exact details of all your references as you go along. If you have a deadline to complete the report, you do not want to be chasing down citations at the very end.

The literature review will help you to refine your original ideas and make them more precise, to be clear about where you want to place your brick. If we go back to our earlier example of oral hygiene, you will find hundreds of articles covering diverse subjects such as oral hygiene marketing products, instructions, routines, courses and so on. Interestingly, if you are a nurse, you will know why oral hygiene is so important, but this is a topic where the best articles are outside the general nursing journals and an example of why wider reading is so important.

If you are not going to be overwhelmed by irrelevant material, you will need to be more specific about your topic so you can reduce the amount of reading to something that is manageable. You may need to go through this process several times until you have a good fit between the topic, the reading, and the time and resources available to you.

WHAT KIND OF LITERATURE REVIEW?

Literature reviews fall broadly into two types: narrative and systematic. *Narrative reviews* have unfairly acquired a bad reputation. They are the traditional way of describing and summarising the state of research in a field on the basis of their author's personal knowledge, reading and networks. As such, they may, of course, be unsystematic, informal and subjective, leading to biased conclusions. However, like all qualitative research, they can also be carried out in a more systematic fashion, selecting exemplary cases for discussion and critical analysis. In practice, this is what most undergraduate and master's level literature reviews look like because of time and resource constraints. However, the development of online citation databases and search tools has made it possible to develop a new form: the *systematic review*. This tries to collect everything that has ever been published on a particular topic, evaluate its quality and aggregate the best of it to produce a firm conclusion. The process of aggregation often involves the use of meta-analysis, where statistical techniques are used to combine different studies in order to produce a more robust conclusion than any individual project could justify on its own. While systematic reviews are often claimed to be more objective, they are very dependent on the quality of the coding of the original papers, which is more problematic in many social sciences than in biomedical research. They are also subject to the biases of the reviewer – the 'objective' hierarchy of evidence that is set beforehand frequently favours poor quantitative studies over well-designed qualitative studies simply because the latter cannot easily be incorporated in the meta-analysis.

———————— FREEING OUR IMAGINATION ————————

If you want to know more about health care systematic reviews, this is a helpful resource: www.ccace.ed.ac.uk/research/software-resources/systematic-reviews-and-meta-analyses

A good example of a systematic review is that of:

Livingston, G., Kelly, L., Lewis-Holmes, E., Baio, G., Morris, S., Patel, N. and Cooper, C. (2014) 'A systematic review of the clinical effectiveness and cost-effectiveness of sensory, psychological and behavioural interventions for managing agitation in older adults with dementia', *Health Technology Assessment,* 18(39). Available at https://doi.org/10.3310/hta18390 (accessed 26/2/20).

For the most part, this chapter recognises that you are unlikely to be able to do a systematic review in the strict sense and will concentrate on describing a systematic approach that can form the basis of a good narrative review.

DEFINING A SEARCH STRATEGY – WHERE DO I START?

Literature searches are nowadays mostly carried out online and you should expect to spend a considerable amount of time logged in, either at home or in a library. You need to become familiar with two kinds of resource: search tools and citation databases. Google Search is probably the most familiar example of a search tool, and The Cumulative Index to Nursing and Allied Health Literature (CINAHL) is the main citation database for nursing. However, there are many other search tools, each

Meta-ethnography is one attempt to develop a more systematic approach to narrative reviewing:

Although the term meta-ethnography parallels meta-analysis, and both approaches share an interest in putting together studies, the similarity ends there. A meta-ethnography synthesises the substance of qualitative research, while meta-analysis synthesises the data.' (Noblitt and Hare, 1988)

Meta-ethnography employs the logic of qualitative analysis discussed in Chapter 9 to compare studies in terms of their similarities, their differences and their cumulative impact. This requires a close reading of the originals to get behind the language that different authors use to describe the observations and interpretations that underlie this. The review process seeks to develop a common language that can assimilate all the studies, either by developing a novel set of terms or by translating the reports of some studies into the language of others. Although they were not explicitly designed in this way, the process is rather like the relationship between the studies of A&E departments described in Chapter 2.

Britten et al. (2002) is an example of the use of meta-ethnography in a health care setting – explaining the meaning of medicines to lay users.

with a different pattern of strengths and weaknesses, and databases for other professional and academic fields that overlap with nursing research. Your library is the best place to advise you on what specific resources are available locally and how to use them. However, we can describe the process of searching a citation database in generic terms because most share a similar logic.

Identify key words in your research problem

The first thing to do is to identify some key words associated with your topic. These are the building blocks for your search strategy. Look at your research question and see how many key words you can create from this. Then review the list and think about other words that are used by your fellow professionals to mean the same thing. Add these terms.

CRITICAL THINKING EXERCISE

Return to your own research problem. Identify all the key words that could be used in your literature search and write them down. Think about any other professional and general terms that might also be used to describe the topic. Add these to the list.

It may help to have a basic plan as shown in Figure 4.1.

Research topic/question
Key words/terms in your topic or question
Alternative words to key terms

Figure 4.1   Template for identifying key words in your research problem

You should end up with something like that shown in Figure 4.2.

Research topic/question
How are the **guidelines** on **oral hygiene** implemented in **different contexts**?
Key words/terms in your topic or question
Oral hygiene, contexts, guidelines
Alternative words to key terms
oral practices, bad oral hygiene, good oral hygiene, oral care, mouth care, mouth hygiene, oral health, oral health care, care of the mouth, oral mouth care, poor mouth care, assessing mouth care, mouth cares, wards, clinical areas, hospital units, clinical units, community, nursing homes, protocols, procedures, practice guidelines etc.

Figure 4.2   Example research problem with key words identified

Note that, at this stage, the search has not been closely tied to the specific research question. You are trying to get broad coverage of the area within which your topic occurs. Within reason, more keywords are better than fewer. The idea is that anything relevant will be somewhere in the first set that you search. You can always narrow this down later but you cannot find things that you have not collected to start with.

The selection process – searching the literature

The actual process of searching the literature is very time consuming. However, if you are organised at the beginning, this can reduce the amount of time you spend on this task. You are trying to balance two possible outcomes:

- Not finding enough papers on the topic.
- Finding too many papers.

The first outcome may, of course, mean that there really are very few papers to be found, but it is more likely that you have not searched widely enough to find the relevant material. Similarly, the second outcome may demonstrate that this is a well-worn topic, but it is equally possible that your search has been so wide that it has swept in a lot of papers that are not very relevant. You may waste a lot of time reading, or skimming, these, to sort out the ones that are actually useful.

Some people adopt structured search frameworks to try to manage this problem. These frameworks can be helpful, although they usually work better with quantitative studies. You do not have to use one, but it is worth knowing that you have the option. There are three common frameworks, which have similar categories:

- PICO – Population/Patient – Intervention – Comparison – Outcome
- PECO – Population – Environment – Comparison – Outcome
- SPIDER – Sample – Phenomenon of Interest – Design – Evaluation – Research Type

PICO was first used in epidemiology and is more commonly associated with quantitative research. Opinions vary about how useful it is for qualitative research. Further details may be obtained from www.ncbi.nlm.nih.gov/pmc/articles/PMC4310146/ (accessed 10/05/20). Table 4.1 illustrates the PICO framework to structure a systematic review.

Table 4.1   Using the PICO framework to structure a systematic review

Population/Patient	**Patient, Population or Problem**
Intervention/Indicator	**Intervention. What treatment do you intend to use?**
Comparator/Control	**What alternatives are there?**
Outcome	**What do you want the result to be?**

You then need to break your inquiry down into component parts, as shown in Table 4.2.

Table 4.2   Components of the PICO framework

Patient/population	Intervention/indicator	Comparator/control	Outcome

PECO works in a similar way, with slightly different headings, as shown in Table 4.3. Again, it is more commonly employed in quantitative studies.

Table 4.3   Using the PECO framework

P	E	C	O
PARTICIPANT PATIENT/POPULATION	**EXPOSURE ENVIRONMENT**	**COMPARISON**	**OUTCOME**
e.g. person with cancer	e.g. city smog or radiation	e.g. the countryside (though there may not always be a comparison)	Compare/ analyse results

SPIDER was developed more specifically for qualitative research. Table 4.4 illustrates its use for a systematic review.

Table 4.4   Using the SPIDER framework for a systematic review

S	PI	D	E	R
SAMPLE	**PHENOMENON OF INTEREST**	**DESIGN**	**EVALUATION**	**RESEARCH TYPE**
e.g. patient	e.g. telemedicine	e.g. technology type	Each case considered individually	Three research types: qualitative, quantitative, and mixed methods

Source: Cooke et al. 2012

Key Point

Collecting articles and writing a good literature review is hard, but it broadens your knowledge about the topic and gives you two generally valuable kinds of experience:

- Knowing how to scan a body of literature on any topic, using a variety of tools, to identify relevant information.
- Applying critical appraisal skills to recognise the best quality studies, which you can regard as the most secure evidence. These skills will transfer into your own practice, even if you do not go on to do more research, and help you to recognise which studies you should use to reflect on, or change, the way you approach your work and your patients.

You may find it useful to refer to the following guide to help find and critically appraise qualitative research articles: http://researchguides.gonzaga.edu/c.php?g=154358&p=1067468 (accessed 26/2/20).

Many published articles offer guidance about the use of search tools. Three studies may be particularly helpful. Flemming and Briggs (2007) compared these search strategies and found that each produced several similar and potentially relevant papers from seven databases. Cooke et al. (2012) found that SPIDER was easier to use when trying to generate search terms and its results were more related to qualitative studies. Methley et al. (2014) compared PICO and SPIDER. They found that PICO generated more hits and was more *sensitive*, meaning that it found a larger number of relevant papers. However, SPIDER searches were more *specific*, meaning that they were better at excluding irrelevant papers. There are, then, no strong grounds for preferring one search strategy over another and you may have your own preferences. If you have time, it is probably worth experimenting to find out which is most useful for the project you are working on. Ultimately it is up to you as to which tool you find most helpful.

Defining search terms: a spider diagram/mind map

If you have a strong visual and spatial component to your thinking and memory, mind mapping can be quite a powerful alternative to structured search frameworks. The spider diagram is one example (see Figure 4.3), where the main idea goes in the centre and your ideas radiate out. Again, it is for you to decide whether it is helpful – our students have been very divided in their opinions!

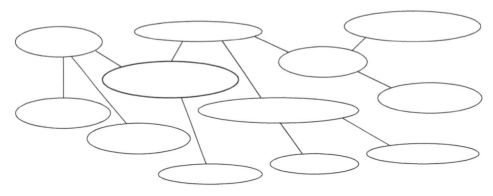

Figure 4.3   A spider diagram/mind map

Searching techniques – Boolean operators

You have identified key words from your research problem/question – and alternative versions of these. Now you need to start searching with a combination of these key and alternative words using Boolean operators.

Boolean operators are simple words (AND, OR, NOT or AND, NOT) used to combine or exclude keywords in a search, resulting in more focused and productive, 'on-target', results. Different search engine or database collections use Boolean operators or coding in different ways: they may require the operator to be typed in capital letters or have special punctuation. The particular phrasing can generally be found in the specific search engine's help screens. Searching in this way saves time and effort by eliminating inappropriate hits without your needing to scan them before you discard them.

For example, use conjunctions to combine or exclude key words in a search:

- AND (xxx AND xxx) finds two terms: narrows results.
- OR (xxx OR xxx) finds either term: widens results.
- NOT (xxx NOT xxx) excludes an area from a search result
- NOT or AND NOT the first term is searched, then any records containing the term after the operators are subtracted from the results.

Truncation

You can use truncation to find alternative endings. You do this by entering the 'root' of the word, then abbreviate with an asterisk or star (★). But be careful not to cut the word too far:

Midwi★ = midwifery / midwife / midwives / midwifing . . .

But it could also be 'midwinter', so extra care is needed!

Controlled vocabularies

A 'controlled vocabulary' is a predetermined set of words and phrases used to index the content of a database, which can then be used to retrieve that content when browsing or searching. This set is known as a 'thesaurus': **MeSH** (**Me**dical **S**ubject **H**eadings), which is widely used in databases of medical journals is an example. You can think of a controlled vocabulary as the database's 'local lingo'. What do you call a soft drink: lemonade, pop, soda, soda pop or coke? What do you wear on your feet: sneakers, trainers or tennis shoes? A controlled vocabulary chooses a single word out of all the possible synonyms.

A database of journal articles will usually be coded using a limited vocabulary of this kind. When you come to search it, you can just look at the thesaurus and choose ready-made search terms. The advantage is that you have a ready-made set of relevant articles. The disadvantage is that you are relying on the quality of the original coding and the terms available may not be a good match for your interests. This is particularly true when you are searching social science databases, where vocabularies are much less standardised. In practice, most searches use some combination of terms from a controlled vocabulary and keywords, either contributed by the original authors of a paper or picked out from its title.

Many databases allow you to save your searches as you progress, especially if you create a personal account. It is always useful to save the details of your search history. This makes it easier to come back later and write about the process by which you collected the body of literature that you are discussing – and how you came to leave some things out! You should also discuss with your library the possible use of software to manage your references. There are several different packages like EndNote, Reference Manager, Zotero and Mendeley. Your institution will probably have a preferred package that you can use free of charge and which will be supported by training materials. If you make this decision when you are doing the literature review, you should be able, with help, to export the search results directly into the citation manager, which will save a lot of work entering everything by hand. In practice, though, if you are doing an undergraduate dissertation, it may not be worth devoting a lot of time and effort to learning these skills and you might just want to keep a separate computer file with a list of documents. Citation managers will reformat references automatically, but if you are keeping your own list, make sure that you have the information you need for your institution's requirements. There are several different systems for formatting references: the world of health sciences often uses one called Vancouver, but social scientists generally prefer Harvard, APA or Chicago. Your library will probably publish a brief guide to the one that you should be using. Make sure you stick to it – some courses will deduct marks if you are not absolutely accurate, and it gives a bad impression of your ability to get other details right.

CRITICAL THINKING EXERCISE

1 Look out for 'review articles'. These are articles, usually written by leading researchers in a particular field, that review the current situation, identifying major themes, limitations and questions that are up to date. This can be a beneficial way of finding other literature and getting a sense of the direction of a field.
2 Select a few articles that interest you and follow up the references they give at the end. This will help you to get a sense of which papers other people have found useful, and will also help you generate a wider breadth of knowledge.

Inclusion and exclusion criteria

Depending on what you are looking for in the literature, at some stage you will need to decide the inclusion and exclusion criteria for anything you find. Your *inclusion* criteria are the features that papers must have if you are going to use them in your review, while *exclusion* criteria are the features that eliminate papers from further consideration. A literature search should be a back-and-forth process between what has previously been published and your own question. You can gradually discard articles that are not relevant to your question and pick up ideas from other people's work that help you to specify what you can most usefully contribute and how this can be done. Your final report should be able to describe how you have come to make the choices you have made in deciding which materials to use.

THE SEARCH

Try to be as systematic as you can. Have a plan! What resources are you going to include in your search? Basically, there are books, journals and web sources.
   Consider:

- Books may provide an introduction, classic text or background information; however, by the time they get to publication, they are invariably out of date. This book was delivered just before the 2020 COVID-19 pandemic (WHO, 2020) and went through production in parallel with it…
- Journals are more focused and specific. They can provide the latest research or primary evidence, although social science journals tend to be published less frequently than medical journals so the findings take longer to appear. However, most journals now put papers online as soon as they have been reviewed, accepted and formatted for publication. Be careful not to confuse these early releases with pre-prints where the author has posted a paper online that they are submitting, planning to submit or thinking about submitting to a journal. These texts have not been reviewed for quality and a significant proportion are never formally published. At your stage, you should probably avoid such sources unless you are very confident about your ability to assess them. You should also beware of predatory journals, where the authors have paid to publish their work and there are very few, if any, quality controls. Your library should be able to help you to recognise these.
- Web sources are easy to maintain, likely to be regularly updated and can provide valid data, although they should always be used critically. Ask yourself who is running a website and why before you take its validity for granted.

Search locations

Your course library will give you access to journals and online databases. This will probably operate through your usual student login when you are on campus, but you may need a special password if you are off campus. There are many databases available, which have been designed in different ways to cover different sorts of material and support different interests. We have listed some of the most important and useful ones in an Appendix at the end of this book.

CASE STUDY SCENARIO

Electronic search tools have transformed literature reviewing – but they have also made it even more important to **have a strategy for searching**. If you have not thought through what you are trying to get out of the literature, you can get seriously lost, miss things or be utterly overwhelmed by the volume of results.
  Think about:

- What is the specific problem, topic or research question that my literature review will help to define?
- What are my inclusion and exclusion criteria?
- What kind of literature review am I conducting? That is, are you looking at issues of theory, methodology or policy, quantitative (e.g. on the effectiveness of a new procedure) or qualitative research (e.g. interviews or observational studies)?
- What is the scope of my literature review? What types of publications am I using (e.g. journals, books, government documents, popular media)?
- What discipline am I working in (e.g. nursing, psychology, sociology, medicine)?

ACTIVE (CRITICAL) READING AND LITERATURE REVIEWS

If you are going to analyse and evaluate research literature, you should also learn how to think and read critically.

Definition

Critical reading is 'the process of carefully and systematically examining [evidence] to judge its trustworthiness, and its value and relevance in a particular context' (CASP, 2018).
  A critique is more focused and tries to assess the actual merits – or otherwise – of a piece of research.

Reading published research reports is commonly described either as 'research review' or 'research critique'. Although these terms are used interchangeably, it should be noted that a review is often simply a description of the literature in a particular field.

All nurses need to develop the skills required for a research critique. You can only decide whether to use the results of a piece of research to influence your professional practice if you can evaluate the report that describes them – and trust the process by which it was produced. Whether or not you ever do another research project of your own, this is a fundamental professional competence, as we noted in Chapter 1.

CRITICAL THINKING EXERCISE

Find and read the following article. It is a good example of a critique of qualitative work.

Depape, A-M. and Lindsay, S. (2015) 'Parents' experiences of caring for a child with autism spectrum disorder', *Qualitative Health Research*, 25(4): 569–83. Available at https://doi.org/10.1177/1049732314552455 (accessed 26/2/20).

Journal articles and other research reports tend to have a similar structure. In many areas of health sciences, the structure is explicitly required by the journal in which it is published. Some social sciences have a more narrative approach, but you can usually identify the same elements.

1   *Reading the abstract*
    o   Does this give you a quick summary and overview of the article?
2   *Reading the introduction* – Does this section:
    o   Identify the purpose of the article?
    o   Review relevant literature?
    o   Identify the research question(s) (or hypotheses) in the research?
    From this section you should know what the researcher wanted to achieve by conducting the research.
3   *Reading the methods section* – This section should tell you:
    o   Who the research participants are?
    o   What kind(s) of data collection tools were used?
    o   How the research study was conducted?
    This section is most important for judging the quality of the research study. You can learn a lot about how to do good research by studying method sections in high-quality, peer-reviewed articles. When you have read the section, you should know precisely how the researcher collected data in order to answer the research questions.
4   *Reading the results section* – This is where qualitative and quantitative articles look most different. However, tables and quotations from interviews or fieldwork notes are just different ways of describing what has been found. The book is primarily about qualitative research so we will not say much about quantitative papers. However, you should develop basic skills in reading them:
    o   Do the reported findings match the abstract?
    o   Do they relate to the questions in the introduction?
    o   Have they been tested for statistical significance?
    o   Has the author got a plausible argument to claim that there is a causal relationship rather than a simple correlation?

A **correlation** is a statistical relationship between two events:

Suppose we observe that a farmyard cockerel crows at the same time as the Sun rises every morning. We cannot say that the Sun *causes* the cockerel to crow. Perhaps there is a third event that links the two, like a member of the farmer's family getting up to feed the chickens so that the crowing is a response to the food not to the sunrise. The sunrise and the crowing are just regular coincidences.

Causation is when one event directly provokes another:

Suppose we examine the cockerel more closely and find light-sensitive receptors in its eye. When light at a certain frequency and intensity falls on these, it triggers an autonomic response in the cockerel's brain that leads to the crowing. We could now say that the sunrise causes the cockerel to crow.

The distinction between correlation and causation does get a lot more complicated than this, but for now it is enough to understand that just because two things often seem to happen at the same time or in the same order, this does not mean you can immediately say that one causes the other. 'Cause' is a strong word in science and needs to be used very carefully.

Qualitative data are harder to summarise, so you will usually be presented with extracts that the author considers to be typical or representative of the data they have collected. You have to decide whether to trust the author on this claim. Your confidence might be increased if they can cite other studies that have presented similar data or if they can show that they have looked in their own data for cases that might not fit. The study author should also be clear about what kind of data they have collected – interviews and observations are not directly comparable. A paper may use both, but should be clear about how each is contributing in a different way to its findings. The commentary on any data extract should also tell you specifically which words or phrases make it evidence of the finding that is claimed. You will find that even quite famous authors are not very good at this – but the reader should not be left to guess what the author was looking at. We shall say more about these issues in Chapter 9 when we come to discuss the analysis of qualitative data.

There are many tools that can help you to critically judge the validity of qualitative research if you are not familiar with it at this stage. One example has been formulated by the Critical Appraisal Skills Programme (CASP, 2017).

When you finish this section of the paper, you should know exactly what the research study has found and have some idea about how solid its evidence is.

5   *Reading the discussion section* – This is the section where the researcher should summarise and explain the results from the study, relate the findings to the literature discussed in the introduction, explain what the practical consequences are, and identify what the next steps/recommendations would be to continue advancing the knowledge in the area.

When you finish this section, you will know what conclusions the researcher portrayed from the research study and what steps were suggested for any future research. Ask yourself if the author goes beyond the conclusions that you thought were reasonable after you read the results section.

6   *Evaluating the Article* – You will do this constantly as you read and think about your article. Use the knowledge you gain from reading to help identify the strengths and weaknesses of the research study. One of the ways you can do this is to generate a table as shown in Table 4.5. Under each theme compare and contrast the findings of different authors and make notes as you go on.

As you become more experienced you may wish to add to or make your own headings or refer to further resources such as Barnett-Page and Thomas (2009). Tables like these are very useful to a reader and help to summarise key studies.

Table 4.5   Example table for identifying the strengths and weaknesses of a research study

Author	Problem	Theories used	Design	Data collection method	Sample size and method	Key points from analysis	Major findings/criticisms

───────────────── FREEING OUR IMAGINATION ─────────────────

Using an online database, download at least ten articles relevant to your research area. You may find that this takes quite a long time, but we recommend that you begin the process of reviewing literature in earnest right at the start of your study, since this will help guide the rest of your reading.

Try to 'actively read' three of these articles to understand them, collating and reviewing their content and argument.

Think about some of the judgements you will be making about the articles. Depending on your reason for reading the paper, you need to bear in mind what you need to focus on. For example, if you are interested in the outcomes of an empirical

(Continued)

(Continued)

study, you would focus on the methods, but if you are reading a literature review article, you should evaluate the search strategy and the range of the material covered. You will also need to check the level and logic of the paper's arguments and ask:

- Do they make sense?
- Are they consistent with the evidence provided?
- Has anything significant been left out?
- Is there is any indication of bias?

APPLYING THE LITERATURE TO YOUR OWN STUDY

The final stage of the literature review process is to write up the results. Remember that the literature review is supposed to tell a story about how you got from your research topic to your research question. Your project should appear to be a logical next step. This is true even if you are just looking at one small problem on one ward – no-one else will have done exactly that. You can find out whether the general consensus of the literature is relevant just here and just now. The introduction to your report should tell the reader quite briefly how you came to choose the topic – perhaps you had some relevant personal experience or perhaps someone suggested that it might be something to look at. The literature review takes the reader onwards to show how you turned that topic into the project that you actually carried out.

> ### Key Point
>
> In practice, especially with postgraduate dissertations, the literature review is often revised again at the very end of the project. This is because research questions are often redefined in the course of qualitative research as the fieldwork reveals more about the topic. A big research project may run over several years, of course, and new material may be published during that time, which affects the direction of the project or which should, at least, be noted in the literature review. However, you could think about a literature review as being like setting up a route on a satnav. You plan your journey from A to B on the best information available but along the way, a key road may be closed for all sorts of reasons and you have to recalculate the route. If you had never planned it in the first place, though, you could not have been sure that you were setting off in more or less the right direction.

The literature review is like a miniature of your whole report. It needs a brief introduction and a description of the methods you used to find relevant literature. The discussion of this literature needs to be organised around themes that will allow you to classify and organise the material, rather than just listing it. You are analysing and evaluating the literature, not just describing it. By the end, you should be able to write a clear justification for your own project. This is the conclusion – and the basis for the next section of your report describing your methods. You will then need to question whether a reader would find your literature review sufficiently comprehensive and useful and if it clearly describes any gap in the literature that your study will ultimately address. If you are not satisfied with the answers to the question, then you need to revise your draft.

——— VIDEO SUPPORT ———

As this book is concerned with qualitative research, a word from David Silverman, a leading sociologist of work and organisations, seems appropriate at this stage in his video *Top Tip: Save Your Literature Review For Last*. You can access the video by visiting this book's online resources: https://study.sagepub.com/dingwallandstaniland.

CHAPTER SUMMARY POINTS

This chapter has discussed how to undertake a literature review and critically judge the resulting articles. It is a chapter that can be followed as required or used as revision or reference depending on the experience of a reader.

Remember, a literature review should:

- Identify appropriate literature and how, or if, others have addressed this problem.
- Be organised around, and related directly to, the thesis or research question.
- Synthesise results into a summary of what is and is not known.
- Identify any theory available to put the current study within a place of importance.
- Contain some judgement about the quality of the published research.
- Identify deficiencies in identified studies which will then provide a rationale for stating how the research problem will fit into the existing literature.
- Formulate questions that need further research.
- Evaluate, select, organise and categorise theories and findings to provide a coherent framework which forms the basis of your research.

In relation to critical writing, you should be able to:

- Present logical arguments which lead into your conclusions.
- Provide sound evidence and reasons to support your argument.

FURTHER READING

There are numerous books offering more detailed advice on literature reviews. These are particularly useful:

Hart, C. (2018) *Doing a Literature Review: Releasing the Research Imagination*. London: Sage.

This puts more emphasis on systematic reviews:

Coughlan, M. and Cronin, P. (2016) *Doing a Literature Review in Nursing, Health and Social Care* (2nd edn). London: Sage.

Systematic reviews in the social sciences are somewhat different from those in the clinical or biomedical sciences. This text is more focused on working with social science literature and databases:

Petticrew, M. and Roberts, H. (2008) *Systematic Reviews in the Social Sciences: A Practical Guide*. Oxford: Blackwell.

If you want to know more about meta-ethnography, a very good overview with some more examples is

Campbell, R., Pound, P., Morgan, M., Daker-White, G., Britten, N., Pill, R., Yardley, L., Pope, C. and Donovan, J. (2011) 'Evaluating meta ethnography: systematic analysis and synthesis of qualitative research', *Health Technology Assessment*, 15(43). Available at https://doi.org/10.3310/hta15430 (accessed 24/2/20).

One of the things we have noted is the need for the literature review to tell a story that justifies your research. This is a short book that may be helpful in developing that skill:

Thomas, R. (2019) *Turn Your Literature Review Into an Argument: Little Quick Fix*. London: Sage.

5
Doing the Right Thing – Ethics in Qualitative Research

> ## Learning Outcomes
>
> At the end of this chapter you will be able to:
>
> - Discuss professional ethics in clinical practice and their relevance to research
> - Apply some basic principles of ethical theory
> - Outline the application of principlism to qualitative research
> - Identify some potential ethical dilemmas in qualitative research

This may seem an unusual way to start a chapter – but we thought we should begin by telling you something that we are not going to do. This chapter is not going to say anything about the *process* of getting through an ethics review. There are two reasons for this silence. The first is that the review process varies so much from one country to another and from one institution to another within a country, that it is just not possible to write a set of instructions that would cover every case. You should expect your course team or project supervisor to guide you through this process or to refer you to specific documents that tell you what you need to do.

The second is that ethics review has taken on a lot of other functions that have blurred its original goals of safeguarding the people who take part in research studies. Some institutions, for example, use it to manage their reputation by blocking research on topics that might be embarrassing for them. Others use it to carry out assessments of the risks to researchers as well as to the research participants. These may be legitimate things for an institution to do but they are not really about ethics.

We want to focus on a different set of issues about how you actually make good decisions for yourself. These are just as important – if not more important – because you will often find that you have to make those decisions on your own, possibly with only a moment to think about them. You are the person who is doing the interview or observing in the field. People expect you to do the right thing there and then, not to hold them up while you phone your supervisor to ask for help. Fortunately, this is something you should be used to as a nurse and the skills involved are not very different from those you would use to make ethical decisions in clinical practice. If you start out from those clinical skills, as we do in this chapter, you have a very solid basis for making sound judgements in research.

—————————————— **VIDEO SUPPORT** ——————————————

At this point you may like to watch *Social Research Ethics – Basic Concepts*, which helps to set the context for this chapter. When it comes to writing up your work, you also need to be aware of current thinking on *publication ethics*, which is the focus of the video *What Can You do to be a **Responsible and Ethical** Researcher?* You can access both of these videos by visiting this book's online resources: https://study.sagepub.com/dingwallandstaniland.

We need to say one other important thing. This is that *not doing research can be unethical.* Many people who write about research ethics seem to forget this and to concentrate solely on the risks to the people who take part. We should always remember that, if we do not do research, we may continue to do things that waste resources, do not deliver their supposed benefits, treat people unfairly, or cause unnecessary pain and suffering.

Research is the key to improving the health of a population, and the services that contribute to that. At the same time, research should not impose a disproportionate risk of harm to those who take part in it.

> ### Key Point
>
> Research ethics are the tools that we use to *balance* risks and benefits – but we should never forget that it is a balance.

PROFESSIONAL ETHICS AND CLINICAL PRACTICE

As a nurse or other health care professional, you are a member of an occupation that has a special legal status. You are allowed to use your expert knowledge and skills in ways that other people are not. In return, you promise not to abuse this privilege by doing things that go against the best interests of your patients or service users. This promise is embedded in the codes of practice that have been adopted by your profession and enforced by its licensing body. If you do not comply with these codes, you may lose your licence to practise.

Ethical codes, however, cannot cover every possible situation that you might find yourself in. Sometimes they do have quite explicit rules, like Section 10 of the Nursing and Midwifery Council *Code* (2018a), which deals with the timely and accurate completion of patient records. More usually, they set out general principles, as in Section 1 of the *Code*, which deals with treating people as individuals and respecting their dignity. When you are faced with a clinical situation where it is not clear how you should act, referring to these principles should steer you in the right direction. Your course will probably have a component on professional ethics where these issues are discussed. One goal for your professional training is likely to be to help you to make many ethical decisions without needing to think about them very much – you just see them as the 'professional' thing to do. You should also find that your workplace is organised in such a way as to encourage you to act in this way. You may not, then, realise how many ethical decisions you are making in the course of your working shift. There are, of course, times when something goes wrong or a new challenge emerges. The 2020 COVID-19 pandemic (WHO, 2020), for example, presented some new ethical problems - and some old ones in new forms. A Rapid Policy Briefing from the Nuffield Council on Bioethics (2020) offered the following guidance:

'Public health measures need to take into account the following ethical principles:

- Interventions should be evidence-based and proportionate. The aim(s) of the interventions being implemented, and the science, values and judgments underpinning those interventions, should be clearly communicated to the public.
- Coercion and intrusion into people's lives should be the minimum possible consistent with achieving the aim sought.
- People should be treated as moral equals, worthy of respect. While individuals may be asked to make sacrifices for the public good, the respect due to individuals should never be forgotten in the way in which interventions such as quarantine and self-isolation are implemented.
- Solidarity is crucial: at the international level, between governments; in support from the state for those bearing the costs of interventions; by businesses in how they exercise their corporate social responsibility; and at the individual level in the way we all respond to the outbreak in day-to-day life.'

If you decide to undertake research in this area, it may be useful to remember these.

These are the moments when you have to go back to the basic principles and ask 'What should I be doing here?' If we look at some of these, we can see that many of them present the same issues that we discuss later in the chapter when we look at ethical choices in research practice.

To help to put this into perspective, below we have chosen five grey scenarios that you might come across in your daily practice that you can think about or discuss with others.

─────────────── FREEING OUR IMAGINATION ───────────────

Balancing patient choice and efficient provision

Suppose you are working on a high-dependency unit. Do you give more attention to a patient who is ready for transfer, alert and wanting you to do things for her, or to a patient who is semi-conscious and unable to ask for help? The first patient is exercising her right to choose when she asks you to meet her needs, but the second patient may benefit more from an extra investment of your time as her advocate in finding out what she might need.

Balancing care quality and efficiency

You are running a focus group with residents of a small NHS treatment unit for young people with anorexia. There is a suggestion that a courtyard could be redeveloped as a garden so that they could grow some of their own food. This might improve their quality of care, but you will have to find money within your budget to pay for the landscaping work. The catering department and the dieticians also complain that it will mean extra complexity and cost for them. Do you just tell the residents that what they have got is as good as it gets with publicly funded health care? Can you justify asking people who pay for the service through their taxes to cover things that would be nice to have rather than essential treatment?

Improving access to care

You are working for a public health department that is responsible for sexually transmitted disease clinics. A clinic is going to have to close because of budget cuts. There are two candidates. One is on the local university campus; it is very busy but most of the people who come are 'worried well' or have problems that could easily be dealt with by the campus pharmacy. The other is in a deprived area where there is a concentration of migrants from countries with high rates of HIV infection. However, the clinic is not particularly busy because the migrants try to avoid contact with public services in case this causes problems for their immigration status. Which clinic should close?

End-of-life care

You are nursing an elderly patient from a minority background who has been admitted from a nursing home with a serious chest infection. The patient has an advanced degree of vascular dementia and the clinical team think that aggressive intervention would be futile and unkind. However, the patient has not declared a wish to avoid resuscitation. There is no Do Not Attempt Resuscitation (DNAR) or advance directive in place. When your team discusses the situation with the patient's family, they are accused of racism. The patient is, they say, being denied treatment because of their ethnicity. If you do not do everything that is theoretically possible, they will take the case to the local media and sue you all. Do you do what you sincerely believe to be the right thing for the patient or follow the family's instructions?

Organ donation

There is a well-documented shortage of organs for transplantation in many countries. You are working on a trauma unit when a young man is brought in with severe head injuries caused in a traffic accident. His organs would be ideal for donation. When you speak to his family, though, it turns out that they are members of a religious group that places great value on the integrity of the body after death. If the cause of death were suspicious, they would accept a coroner's order for a postmortem, but otherwise the body must be buried intact. The country where you are working has a law that presumes the consent of the deceased to the donation of their organs unless they have previously registered an individual objection. The clinical team could just go ahead and remove the organs, whatever the family says. Would the clinicians be right to do so?

We are sure you could add other, perhaps more everyday, examples. As you probably realise, though, from these cases, ethical questions rarely have a single correct answer. People can, and do, reasonably disagree about what weight to give to the competing claims in any of these situations. They cannot, however, avoid making a decision. Even putting off a decision is a decision of a kind. What usually matters, then, is the clarity of the thinking that leads them to that choice. Ethical theory is intended to be a tool you can use to get things clearer.

INTRODUCING ETHICAL THEORIES

As with anything that academics are involved with, there is a large and complicated literature on ethical theory. We are not going to cover everything here; if you need to, you can refer to other reading, but we will cover just enough to help you navigate the practical choices you may need to make in the course of your data collection and analysis.

> **Key Point**
>
> Most ethical theories fall into one or other of two traditions:
>
> - *Consequentialism* – taking the consequences of our actions into considera-
>   tion. The most familiar type of consequentialism in health care is *utilitarianism*.
> - *Deontology* – basing our actions on a set of principles or duties. Deontol-
>   ogy lays out a set of duties or principles which are the criteria to be used in
>   advance to decide whether or not an action is moral or ethical.

Consequentialism focuses on the outcomes of our actions. We only find out for certain whether or not we did the right thing in retrospect. In practice, of course, since we have to act first, before we can have an outcome, we try to predict the result and then assess whether it would be right or wrong.

Utilitarianism is particularly associated with two 19th-century philosophers called Jeremy Bentham and John Stuart Mill. Its leading contemporary advocate is Peter Singer. They argued that we should always choose to act in ways that bring the greatest benefit to the greatest number of people. The problem here is one of calculation. How do we measure benefits? How do we balance a large benefit to a small number of people against a small benefit to a large number of people? How do we offset benefits and harms? Peter Singer, for example, has suggested that we need not consider people with severe learning disabilities as fully human beings (Singer and Kuhse, 1985). We might, then, be justified in killing them so we could use their organs for transplantation. The death of one less-than-human person might prolong the lives of a number of fully human people. This would bring a greater benefit to society than preserving the 'donor's' limited existence and allowing the potential recipients of their organs to die.

You might recognise a similar argument in the 'Improving access to care' scenario where you had to choose between serving a large number of students with minor STIs and a small number of migrants with serious STIs. Utilitarianism is often quite provocative in this way and there are relatively few people who would press the case as far as Peter Singer does. It is, though, helpful to think about where such an argument leads to, especially if you are going to justify a position that stops somewhere short of that conclusion. If you are not going to maximise benefit (or minimise harm), why not? Do you have good reasons to stop short? Those reasons are likely to be *deontological*. As stated previously, this kind of theory lays out a set of duties or principles which are the criteria to be used in advance to decide whether or not an action is moral or ethical. It is not interested in consequences so much as in whether the action is inherently the right thing to do. If it does not fit these criteria, we should not do it, regardless of the benefits that it might bring.

> **Key Point**
>
> There are two main foundations for deontological theories. One looks to
> *religion*, while the other is more *secular*.

All major faiths have developed some kind of statement about what it means to be human and the rights and duties that go with that. Ideas such as *human dignity*, for example, take their inspiration from the principle that all human beings have some kind of intrinsic value in the eyes of their Creator and are entitled to have this respected. Whatever the potential benefits, there are some things that you just should not do to people. You might recognise this in the organ donor example. Particular faith groups within Christianity, Judaism and Islam share strong beliefs about the integrity of the dead body. It is simply wrong to open this up and remove parts, even if others benefit. In rare cases, such as suspected murder, members of such groups may defer to the state's interest in investigating crime by accepting autopsies. However, in democratic societies, the state is generally reluctant to enforce this interest unless there is a clear reason to do so.

Since the late 18th century, a secular version of this approach has developed, which is today most recognisable in the form of claims about *human rights*. These rights do not flow from a divine source but simply from membership in the community of humans. In a modern form, they are the basis of the first two clauses of the *United Nations Universal Declaration of Human Rights*:

Article 1. All human beings are born free and equal in dignity and rights. They are endowed with reason and conscience and should act towards one another in a spirit of brotherhood.

Article 2. Everyone is entitled to all the rights and freedoms set forth in this Declaration, without distinction of any kind, such as race, colour, sex, language, religion, political or other opinion, national or social origin, property, birth or other status. Furthermore, no distinction shall be made on the basis of the political, jurisdictional or international status of the country or territory to which a person belongs, whether it be independent, trust, non-self-governing or under any other limitation of sovereignty. (United Nations, 1948)

Similar statements can be found in most such declarations. However, a consensus about the document does not always lead to a consensus about what it means in practice. We have already noted, for example, that some writers, like Peter Singer, question who counts as a human being. Apart from his position on people with severe learning disabilities, Singer also argues that the capacities of some great apes may be such as to entitle them to be considered as having the same rights as humans. Clearly, there might also be debate about what a word like 'dignity' means in practice. You might think of the above 'End-of-life care' scenario here. Which is more conducive to human dignity – aggressive intervention to prolong life for a short period or peaceful death as a result of the infection?

In the field of health care, these two streams, consequentialism and deontology, are often combined in what is known as *principlism*, an approach originally developed by Beauchamp and Childress in their 1979 book, *Principles of Biomedical Ethics* – this book is now in its eighth (2019) edition. They identified four ethical principles: autonomy, beneficence, non-maleficence (to do no harm) and justice. Two of these principles, autonomy and justice, are broadly deontological, and two, beneficence and non-maleficence, are broadly consequentialist. Let us look at each of these in more detail.

Definition

Autonomy is the basic right of any person to make their own decisions about their own lives. As such, it is a deontological principle. In practice, however, it may not be straightforward to operate. The principle assumes that the person making the decision is fully informed about the likely costs and benefits and is competent to assess those for themselves.

In many health care contexts, professionals may be better informed than patients, and patients may lack the capacity to make decisions. A patient may be unconscious or have some kind of cognitive impairment: a small child, someone with a learning disability or a mental health problem, or a person with dementia. If this principle is pushed too far, it may also collide with the principle of justice: does an individual have the right to everything they might desire from a health care system even if this means that others who are less competent or articulate then get less than they might need? It is, however, an important challenge to the idea that health care professionals always know best and are entitled to act in a paternalist way.

Definition

Beneficence is the idea that any action should, if possible, benefit the people who are affected by it. It is a consequentialist principle in that it focuses on the intended outcome of the action. We do not give medications to people 'just to see what happens', for example.

Again, there are complications because we may intend actions to be beneficial but we cannot always be certain that this will be the outcome. A surgeon may carry out extensive tests and scans before operating to remove a tumour, but when she gets inside the body of the patient, she may discover that the cancer has disseminated so far that it cannot be removed. She intended to act for the patient's benefit, but that outcome could not be achieved. This does not mean that it was unethical to begin the surgery in the first place.

Definition

Non-maleficence is a consequentialist principle, introduced partly because of the difficulties of establishing beneficence in advance. What it says is that, even if we cannot be certain about the benefit of our actions, we can at least try to be sure that we will do no harm. Florence Nightingale anticipated this principle in *Notes on Nursing* (1860): 'The very first requirement in a hospital is that it should do the sick no harm.'

In most circumstances, this is an easier test to meet than that of beneficence, but some uncertainty cannot be avoided. You may give a patient an antibiotic from the penicillin family to treat a minor infection without being sure whether it is bacterial or viral, but the patient suddenly displays an unexpected allergic reaction. You thought that you would do no harm, even if the infection was viral and the antibiotic would be ineffective, but it turned out that the patient had a sensitivity that neither they nor you had suspected.

Justice is the other deontological principle and refers to an obligation to treat people fairly and equally. You should not favour some individuals or groups over others or, alternatively, discriminate against individuals or groups. This may sound straightforward but it is also quite complex in practice. 'Fairness' might mean treating everyone in the same way – but this might actually discriminate against people who come from a different background in terms of language or culture or whose capacity is otherwise limited. Being fair might actually mean treating people equitably, varying your approach and treatment to try to ensure that everyone with similar needs gets to achieve a similar outcome. There is often some tension between justice and autonomy.

Definition

You will find other approaches discussed in bioethics textbooks, particularly an approach called 'virtue ethics', which has become increasingly influential. This is partly in response to some of the limitations of principlism and the way in which it has lent itself to checklist approaches in clinical practice. However, we are not writing a bioethics textbook and you will find principlism sufficient for the issues you are likely to come across in the kind of research project this book is designed to support. We would stress, though, the importance of not treating the four principles as a set of tick boxes. It is better to see them as a series of questions that you should ask yourself when you are designing a project or when you are presented with an ethical problem in the course of your research. If you had to, how would you justify your actions if someone asked you each of these questions?

PRINCIPLISM AND QUALITATIVE RESEARCH

Key Point

Qualitative research is often thought to raise difficult ethical problems. In fact, it is less that the ethical problems are particularly difficult, or even specific to qualitative methods, than that it does not easily fit into the processes used by ethics regulators.

Quantitative researchers generally do more design and planning up front. This means they can submit much more specific proposals for approval. Survey work, for example, is highly bureaucratised, whether it is done by telephone, online or face to face. Regulatory controls can be built into its internal management systems. Qualitative research, however, particularly when using observational methods, is less suited to regulation-in-advance or *anticipatory regulation* (Murphy and Dingwall, 2001) and depends heavily on the researcher's immediate ethical judgments as problems arise. Nevertheless, some potential problems can be thought about ahead of time and, as Murphy and Dingwall showed, principlism can be a useful way of identifying them. They approached the principles in a slightly different order, which better reflects their application to research rather than clinical practice.

Key Point

The principles of *non-maleficence* and *beneficence* are more closely linked in a research context because it is often the case that people who participate in research will not get a personal, direct and immediate benefit from it. Their participation contributes to a more distant goal of improvements for others who may be in a similar position to themselves.

Of course, this is not always the case. If you are studying patient experiences in a particular ward or clinic, for example, you may be able to introduce improvements quite quickly. Alternatively, you may be studying people who have a chronic condition, where their relationship with health professionals may last long enough for them to see personal benefits. However, the main focus in planning qualitative research is usually on demonstrating that it will not harm the people who take part in it.

What kinds of harm might arise? Murphy and Dingwall show that possible harms may be short-term and long-term, direct and indirect, but that there is nothing that compares with the immediate potential damage that can be done by administering an experimental drug (Hedgecoe, 2014). There are also complex judgements involved in assessing whether a reaction is, or is not, harmful.

Key Point

Research participants may experience anxiety, stress, guilt and damage to self-esteem during data collection.

In observational fieldwork, participants may form close relationships with the observer, resulting in an experience of loss when the study is completed and the observer withdraws. Informants in interviews may feel embarrassed – about the opinions they hold, or because they do not hold opinions on matters about which the interviewer expects them to have opinions. They may be provoked to feel discontented about things that they have previously taken for granted: an interview about who does what around the home might lead a woman to recognise how unfairly tasks are shared, for example. Is this necessarily harmful? Will she still be upset when she has had more time to reflect, or will she be grateful that the issue was raised?

CONFIDENTIALITY, ANONYMITY AND PRIVACY

REFLECT ON PRACTICE

It is very important to ensure that the confidentiality, anonymity and privacy of participants are maintained in your research. This can be difficult to achieve in qualitative research if you are conducting face-to-face interviews, focus groups or participant observation. It is essential to assure the participant that the original data will be only be seen by yourself, your project supervisor, and, possibly, an external examiner, unless you are legally required to disclose it (Hughes, 2018).

This obligation can present nurses with some difficult dilemmas if they observe unsafe practice or receive information that someone is at risk of harm. The basic ethics of field research may conflict with the ethical duties set out in a professional code. If you think this might happen in your project, you should discuss your options with your supervisor. You should certainly not disclose information without their agreement and support.

Some potential harms only appear further down the track. Research participants are often dissatisfied with what is written about them. In a way this is inevitable because each one has a partial perspective on the setting that is being studied, while the researcher is trying to show how those partial perspectives fit together as a whole. When all the parts come together, well-intentioned actions may actually appear to be damaging. There is, too, often concern about the consequences of publishing accounts of the ways in which lower-status people make their lives and jobs more comfortable. Describing how nurses use fetching supplies in a hospital to create space for smoking breaks, for example, may not be used to understand the need for breaks but as a way to eliminate them and intensify the nurses' workload.

While it is not likely to be immediately relevant to your studies, once research is published, it is also open to being abused by the mass media. Your carefully balanced writing about the problems faced by a stigmatised group, like people with HIV, in accessing health care may be used to denounce their 'irresponsible behaviour' and the demands created by its consequences.

How do we deal with this? Traditionally, social scientists have placed great stress on promising research participants that they will remain anonymous in any published work and that the original data will be kept strictly confidential and shared only with people trusted by the researcher. This is not an institutional promise: it is a personal ethical commitment that has been made by qualitative researchers ever since the beginnings of such work in the 1840s. It is what we do. However, this commitment has come under pressure in recent years by demands for data sharing and greater accessibility by other researchers in general. This movement has been driven mainly by people working in biomedical research, where it is relatively easy to anonymise data, as it is in much quantitative social science. However, it is often impracticable to edit field notes or interview transcripts in ways that protect the identities of research participants while still being useful for other researchers. They simply contain too much detail of times, places and lives: if this is removed, they become unintelligible. You are unlikely to encounter this concern in a student project but you should be careful that the original data are only shared with people who need to know, like your supervisor or adviser, or people you trust.

Key Point

You should also use pseudonyms in your reports or dissertations and consider altering non-relevant details. Even so, you cannot guarantee that people will not be recognisable to themselves and those closest to them: 'Did I really say that?' is not an uncommon reaction. You should be careful about giving *absolute* assurances to your research participants.

STORAGE OF DATA

Always bear in mind that there are legal requirements under the Data Protection Act 2018 and the General Data Protection Regulation 2018 which are intended to prevent unauthorised people from accessing information about individuals (see www.legislation.gov.uk/ukpga/1998/29/section/33, accessed 27/2/20).

Your university should have policies and practices in place to manage these requirements. These vary somewhat, but you will normally have to satisfy ethics reviewers that any data you collect will be stored securely, as defined locally. At a minimum, you should use password-protected files for the data and store hard copy in a locked filing cabinet. If your university offers secure cloud storage for data, you should use that rather than having a copy on your own laptop, where it might be at risk of getting lost or stolen. You could back this up on a flash drive or an external hard drive, which has password protection and is kept in a secure place.

PERSONAL RISK AND DISTRESS

One other topic that we could add here, although it is not strictly a matter of research ethics, is the level of personal risk and distress that you should accept. It is not just research participants who get upset by qualitative research. Although many students, and established researchers, choose topics because they have a strong personal investment in them, the data collection can then be quite stressful. This emotional engagement may have implications for the analysis of your data – which we shall come to later in this book – but you should always try to think about how you will cope with people telling you sad stories in interviews or resenting your presence in the field.

CASE STUDY SCENARIO

Suppose your grandfather died from prostate cancer and you decide to study the experiences of men with that condition. How will you deal with what they tell you in interviews - which may reveal things your grandfather experienced but chose to shelter his family from?

You may place yourself physically at risk too. One PhD student supervised by RD interviewed men who had been violent towards their former partners. In partnership with her supervisors, she identified places to interview them where there would be other people around in the building and arranged a phone-in system with a friend to establish that she had returned home safely. On the other hand, Staci Newmahr (2011), whose work on an SM club we have already mentioned, allowed herself to be whipped within the safety limits established by the community of members. She assessed the risk and made the choice, trusting in the conventions established within her field site, and the way people were expelled from the club if they became too violent. Anthropologists, particularly when working in developing countries, have long accepted real risks of physical and sexual assault. You should always weigh up the risks to yourself, and how you might manage them, as you choose and design a project. Beneficence and non-maleficence apply to you too!

Key Point

Autonomy recognises that people can be wronged as well as harmed by research. If you accept the deontological view that people have certain rights just because they are human, then you need to recognise that these might be infringed.

Research can, in particular, encroach on rights to privacy, respect and self-determination. There is, for example, a long-established debate about the ethics of covert research, where the researcher does not tell the participants who she is and what she is doing. Critics point out that this does not respect the autonomy of the participants and their right to decide for themselves whether or not to take part in the study. The research may invade their private space, or at least space that they think of as private. The conventional response to this problem is *informed consent*, which should not be confused with getting a consent form signed. Although your university or hospital may require them, consent forms are mostly documents designed to protect the organisation (Wynn and Israel, 2018).

As a researcher your ethical responsibility is to ensure that research participants understand the potential consequences of co-operating with you. Unfortunately, this is not completely straightforward. There are four main reasons for this:

1   You do not want to contaminate your research site. If you tell people too much about what you are looking for, you may influence their behaviour or their answers to your interview questions. You also have to think about explaining the research in terms that they will understand and be willing to go along with. You cannot send the participants to the classes on research methods that you have attended. In order to be *persuasive*, your account of the research may also be *evasive*.

2   Your research participants are unlikely to understand your research in the way that you do. They will not have been to the same classes in research methods or thought about their lives as objects of study in the way that you have. In some cases, your participants may have an impaired capacity to understand or be in a position where they cannot refuse your approach. You will often find such people described as members of *vulnerable* groups, and research ethics regulators tend to have checklists to identify them. Vulnerability, however, is really something that goes with a situation rather than with a person. With sufficient forethought, you can explain what research means both to children and to adults with a range of mental health problems, learning disabilities, dementia and similar limitations. Simply excluding people because they are assumed to be vulnerable violates one aspect of the ethical principle of justice: that everyone has a right to participate in research that may potentially benefit them or people like them.

3   As we have seen, it is inherent in many qualitative research designs that you do not know exactly how the research is going to unfold until you start doing it. As you come to understand the research site or research topic better, your questions and focus may shift, leading you to talk to people or go into places that you had not expected to. We do not want to make too much of this, because we think that a well-designed project will anticipate many of these possibilities. Nevertheless, there is always an element of *uncertainty*: you cannot inform people about your plans because you do not know what those are.

4   Particularly in observational research, there are always likely to be people coming and going on the margins of the group you are studying. RD has described these people as the 'spear-carriers' – people who may fill up the stage in a play but do not have a speaking part (Dingwall, 1980). You may be able to introduce yourself – but this may not always be possible or desirable, if you are trying to minimise your impact.

For example, when RD was studying health visitors, he always left them to make the introductions when doing a home visit. He insisted on being identified as a researcher, rather than as a student or other companion, but left the health visitors to determine how best to integrate the request for access into the flow of the visit.

————————————— **FREEING OUR IMAGINATION** —————————————

Informed consent

Remember: Typically, at the start of qualitative research, consent is both tentative and limited. The researcher's access to sensitive aspects of the setting may be restricted. Over time, as trust builds between a researcher and their hosts, access may be granted to previously restricted areas or interactions. However, such access is rarely guaranteed and depends upon the researcher's personal capacity for sustaining their hosts' goodwill and co-operation. Such co-operation can be, and sometimes is, withdrawn.

The term 'informed consent' means the participant has been *fully informed* as to the nature and intended purpose of the research. In qualitative research, this is often a dynamic process, rather than the one-off reading of a letter or signing of a form. The researcher can tailor information to their hosts' level of understanding and to the particular context in which they are currently working. This information can be extended or adapted as the fieldwork moves into new contexts or encounters new informants. This places heavy demands on the researcher's integrity, in giving fair, accurate and honest answers to the questions they may be asked, without compromising their ability to carry out the project in a rigorous and valid fashion.

COVERT RESEARCH

Although many ethics regulators do not like it, covert research can sometimes be justifiable. You might be doing research in a public place, for example, where there is no reasonable expectation of privacy. Suppose you were interested in what office workers ate at lunchtime, for example. Do they bring food from home, or buy healthy options, or do they prefer to buy snacks high in sugar or fat? In many cities, these workers will sit outside in a public square to eat their lunch so you could walk round and observe what they were eating and what they had packed in lunchboxes. You could also map the interactions between them. Do they eat on their own or in groups? Does this make any difference to what they are eating? Similar arguments have been made about social media. You might want to look at tweets using a particular hashtag as evidence for the way people think about some health issue – but remember that Twitter's terms of service restrict research use. There have also been successful and important covert studies of some stigmatised or marginalised groups. However, these do involve risks to the researcher that are not really appropriate at the level of this textbook.

> **Key Point**
>
> The really important thing here is to treat people with respect and to be as honest and truthful with them as you feel you reasonably can be without undermining the research.

Both authors have had students who thought that it would make their projects much easier if they did not tell people what they were doing. They assumed that covert research would be easier. Except where you are studying people in public places, it is not. If it is not to violate the autonomy principle, the level of deception involved in covert research requires stronger justifications than most student projects could argue. We would not say that it should never be done, nor that researchers are obliged to explain their projects to participants at the level of a university seminar or an academic conference. Autonomy is not an absolute right, but it is one that matters very much.

Definition

In the context of qualitative research, **justice** is usually taken to mean 'taking sides'. Perhaps researchers have a special obligation to listen to people whose voices are often ignored and to speak on their behalf? In what is sometimes called *standpoint* research, the investigator approaches the topic with a commitment to an analysis in certain ethical or political terms, by reference to issues of class, gender, race, sexuality or whatever.

We are not so sure about this aspect of justice within qualitative research. There are three particular dangers:

1   Research simply illustrates what the researcher, and those who think like her, already know. It is simply there to provide some nice anecdotes that make their claims more persuasive. However, it does not necessarily persuade anyone who is sceptical about qualitative research to start with. As the British sociologist Ann Oakley (1998) has commented, the feminist cause may, in practice, be advanced much more by disinterested research than by obviously fitting data to a prior standpoint.

2   By claiming to speak for a silenced group, the researcher may actually silence them further, especially if she only repeats claims that support her own previous position. This can be a problem with certain kinds of research that are closely linked to community action. People have their own voices and sometimes they say things that standpoint researchers do not want to hear. Similarly, by excluding a supposedly vulnerable group, the researcher may actually be increasing their vulnerability by denying them the opportunity to benefit from research that describes their disadvantages and analyses the causes.

3 By focusing on underdogs, the researcher may fail to understand the social processes that actually placed them into this position. Indeed, this is often taken for granted in the standpoint analysis. For example, it is widely claimed that doctors dominate consultations with patients just because they ask a lot of questions. When you think about it, though, why wouldn't they? The patient has come because they have a problem they cannot solve on their own and the doctor has to ask questions to find out what that problem is. This is just what happens when one person in an interaction has more expertise than the other (Pilnick and Dingwall 2011).

Key Point

We think that it is important not to confuse *research* and *advocacy*. This is a classic position in social science, which was defined by the German sociologist Max Weber in two lectures he gave in 1917 and 1919 (Gerth and Mills 1970: 77–158). It is one thing to look impartially at the world and another to make judgements about the morality of what you observe and how you should act in the light of what you know.

Of course, it can be very hard to separate 'facts' and 'values' but, trying to do so – and certainly recognising when you are doing one and when the other – is a valuable discipline. Murphy and Dingwall (2003) describe it as a 'regulative ideal', something that you should try to achieve, even if you sometimes fall short. In their view, justice should be understood as what they call 'fair dealing'. By this they mean that, in principle, everyone the researcher comes across should be treated equally and with equal seriousness of purpose to understand how they come to think and act in the way that they do. There should be equal attention and sympathy for both obvious villains and obvious heroes or heroines (Dingwall, 1992).

If you want to understand a social, organisational or professional problem, you need, as far as possible, to understand both those who are its victims and those who contribute to the social, economic and cultural structures that advantage some people more than others. You do not just look at the underdogs – you also look at the top dogs and at the people in the middle, who we might term 'lapdogs'. Of course you may have different levels of access to these groups, but your ethical obligation is to try to represent them fairly and impartially in reporting your study, even if you then go on to pass judgement on some of them.

POTENTIAL ETHICAL DILEMMAS IN QUALITATIVE RESEARCH

This has been quite an abstract chapter, so we are going to finish with two cases, based on real examples, for you to think through.

CASE STUDY SCENARIO 1

You are interested in studying how children play with each other outside hospitals, in order to compare this with play on a children's ward where you are working. Perhaps you can improve the experience of your child patients if you can make their play more 'normal'.

You arrange access to a nearby private day nursery, which uses the converted outbuildings of the farmhouse where the owner lives. You start on a programme of half-day visits to collect data for your degree project. After a few of these, you realise that the owner's adult son, who seems to you to have some kind of moderate learning disability or other mental health problem, is regularly taking some of the children over to the house in order to give them a bath. When the children return, you can see no obvious signs of abuse or distress but this does not seem like best practice in terms of safeguarding.

What should you do?

CASE STUDY SCENARIO 2

You are observing how phlebotomists manage taking blood samples from confused patients on an elderly care ward. You want to find out whether there are particular features of the interaction between the phlebotomist and the patient that could be changed so that the patients respond more calmly. One particularly confused patient knocks the cannula out of the phlebotomist's hand, and it falls on the floor. She mutters something about the five-second rule, picks it up and is about to try again to insert it into the patient's vein.

What should you do?

What would we do?

In the first of these cases, there is no immediate urgency because there is no indication that the children involved are distressed. You should certainly discuss the case with your supervisor, who will probably want to take further advice from the university administration and, perhaps, from their lawyers. This may take some days and you should continue your fieldwork as normal, if you feel able to. However, we would expect your concern to be taken up officially by the university. This may involve a meeting between your supervisor and the owner of the nursery or it may involve a formal report to the social services department, which will license the nursery's operation. Although you will be breaching the terms of your access to the nursery and any promises you made about the confidentiality of your data, you have a clear *professional obligation* here. (This case is based on one that RD dealt with as a head of department, which was eventually taken to social services. Their investigation did not establish that the children were being abused but they found other grounds to close down the nursery.)

In the second case, you must make an immediate decision about whether to step in and insist the phlebotomist uses a new cannula. This may be a finer judgement in balancing your professional duty against the value of maintaining good relations with the phlebotomists you are observing. While this is not best practice, because of the risks of contamination, those risks are very low and you may think that there is a greater benefit in not calling out the phlebotomist in that moment but perhaps quietly asking her later why she acted in that way. By showing that you are not shocked by such events, perhaps you will get to see more of them and be able to get a better understanding of how they come to occur.

In the original case, the observer was a very experienced professor of nursing who was observing a student for a research project. Her decision was to take over the whole procedure and insert a new cannula herself.

KS, as a nurse, would have stopped the procedure, thinking of her professional duty of care for the wellbeing of individual patients.

RD, as a sociologist, would probably have let it go, recognising the mistake but not feeling a professional obligation to challenge it there and then. He would have put more weight on the potential collective benefit from retaining the trust of the phlebotomist and learning more about how she came to think this was acceptable practice.

WHO DO YOU THINK WOULD BE RIGHT?

There may seem to be a lot to think about when you are collecting data and, as the last phlebotomist case illustrates, some questions may not have a single correct answer. This is as it should be – research comes with both costs to individual participants and benefits for a wider community. Different researchers, like RD and KS, may quite legitimately strike a different balance between those costs and benefits. What matters is that they have thought through their choice and can justify it if asked to do so. However, if you start out by intending to treat the people who take part in your research in the way you are expected to treat your patients, you will not go far wrong.

CHAPTER SUMMARY POINTS

In this chapter we have discussed various professional ethics in clinical practice and their relevance to research, applied some basic principles of ethical theory, described and outlined the application of principlism, and reviewed some potential ethical dilemmas in qualitative research.

The main points to remember are:

- The ethical issues raised by qualitative research are very similar to those that you regularly meet in clinical practice.
- Ethical dilemmas will inevitably arise in qualitative research, as they do in clinical practice.
- You should always seek advice from your project supervisor or another appropriate person before beginning any research.

Because they vary so much, we have *not* discussed specific local requirements for obtaining ethics approval to carry out research. You *must* read those that are produced where you are and comply with them. Your course team or supervisor should be able to direct you to these.

FURTHER READING

The most comprehensive guide to bioethics is:

Beauchamp, T. and Childress, J. (2019) *Principles of Biomedical Ethics* (8th edn). New York: Oxford University Press.

If you are mainly concerned with issues of research ethics, you may find these more useful:

Israel, M. (2014) *Research Ethics and Integrity for Social Scientists: Beyond Regulatory Compliance* (2nd edn). London: Sage.

Kara, H. (2018) *Research Ethics in the Real World: Euro-Western and Indigenous Perspectives*. Bristol: Policy Press.

Nuffield Council on Bioethics (2020) Ethical considerations in responding to the COVID-19 pandemic www.nuffieldbioethics.org/assets/pdfs/Ethical-considerations-in-responding-to-the-COVID-19-pandemic.pdf (accessed 08/05/2020).

6

Observing People

Learning Outcomes

At the end of this chapter you will be able to:

- Define observational research
- Describe the different roles that observers may take when studying the social processes involved in modern health care
- Identify the strengths and weaknesses of observational research
- Recognise field notes as a foundation of using observational research as data
- Appreciate the potential of audio and video recording to replay and review observations in different ways.

This is the point at which we start to talk about actually *doing* qualitative research. Not before time, you might think, although we hope that we have shown you how important it is to have a solid foundation of understanding what you are going to do before you start undertaking it! This chapter, and the two that follow, will look at how to collect qualitative data through observation, interviews and the study of documents and artefacts or, if you prefer, through 'hanging out', 'asking questions' and 'reading the papers'. Collectively, these methods are sometimes described as *ethnography*, although Howard Becker (2017: 44), one of the most influential qualitative researchers of the last sixty years, has argued that we should stop using this term. He thinks that it leads researchers to be unacceptably vague about exactly what they have done to produce their data. We have previously been guilty of this ourselves, but we think his argument is persuasive, so we are not going to use that term here, unless it occurs in something we are quoting. When you write about your methods, be specific.

We are going to start by focusing on *observation*. We have decided to do this because observation is widely accepted as the 'gold standard' for qualitative research. You may find more studies using interviews and documents because they are generally quicker and cheaper to carry out, and they are easier to regulate. However, you should really see these as second-best choices, to be used when, for one reason or another, it is not possible to achieve your goals by an observational study. Observational studies are likely to be more difficult for a time following the COVID-19 pandemic. There are, however, ways to carry them out on online chat groups or using audio or video for remote observations so that you can learn the key skills for the most important type of qualitative methods.

We begin by defining observational methods and describing how you would do them in the traditional way, as a human being taking some part in the situation you are studying. Later in the chapter, we shall discuss the increasing use of audio and video recording to capture the same sorts of events and the new opportunities created by their capacity to provide repeated action replays.

OBSERVATION

All health care professionals use the basic skills of observation in their everyday work. A community nurse, for example, may visit an older person at home to change the dressing on a leg ulcer. In the course of performing this task, the nurse will also be assessing that person's general level of physical and mental wellbeing, observing the conditions of the house and its furnishings, and the state of the kitchen or bathroom. If there are other people – family, friends or neighbours – present, the nurse can observe how they interact with the patient. This yields information about the older person's general mental state and the social support available to them. Nurses collect information through their five senses. They then use their professional knowledge and experience to draw inferences from that information and reach a conclusion about what they should do next for, or with, that person in that context. This process is sometimes described as a nurse's 'instinct', but it is actually the mobilisation of professional knowledge and experience that have become tacit, as we described in Chapter 1.

Observational research in the social sciences uses the observer's senses in exactly the same way. The main differences lie in the rigour with which the findings from those senses are documented and in the use to which the information is put. Observation is hanging out in a systematic and purposeful way. Where the community nurse is interested in the specifics of the case, the social scientist, or the nurse doing social science, is interested in what *this instance* can tell us about cases *of this kind*. We shall come back to the question of what 'of this kind' means in Chapter 9. For now, we want to focus on how data are collected.

CASE STUDY SCENARIO

If, as a nurse, you cringe when you see some of the practices that are depicted in medical dramas or soaps on television, you have already started to do observational research. You are noticing differences between your own experiences and a dramatist's reconstruction of similar events. If you then go on to discuss what you have seen with other students or colleagues, you are beginning to develop an analysis that defines the differences and attempts to explain them. You may also notice new things about your own practice - things that you normally do without thinking or noticing until you suddenly see someone else not doing them. Now that you have noticed them, you can ask whether you should be doing them – remember our example of the old-style sister and her polished ward in Chapter 1.

THE PROCESS OF OBSERVATIONAL RESEARCH

At its most basic, observational research involves a social scientist, or a nurse acting as a social scientist, placing him/herself into some situation and recording what happens there. This is often described as 'going into the field' and making 'field notes'.

In its most inclusive sense, **fieldwork** is simply research conducted in natural social settings, in the actual contexts in which people pursue their daily lives. The fieldworker ventures into the worlds of others in order to learn first-hand how they live, how they talk and behave, what captivates and distresses them. Whether it is the classic anthropologist trekking across the world to live with some remote tribe, the urban ethnographer moving into some hidden segment of the modern city, the participant observer sharing in and observing the lifeways of a local community or joining the rush-hour commute to study the lifeworlds of modern bureaucrats, the fieldworker's first commitment is to enter the ongoing worlds of other people to encounter their activities and concerns first hand and close up. (Emerson et al., 2011: 1)

Definition

There are some refinements to this. Where nursing students are concerned, 'the field' may be a work site that they normally participate in, which poses some special challenges. Some studies may use remote methods – studying behaviour in a waiting area with the help of CCTV footage or having an online feed from a teleconsultation – so that the observer is not physically present. While field notes were traditionally taken by hand, and often still are, they may now be supplemented or replaced by audio or video recording. What is crucial is that the situation has not been created for the purposes of the research. Watching people interacting in a waiting area on CCTV is not the same as observing an artificial game through a one-way mirror in a psychology laboratory. There are some fine distinctions: a psychology laboratory could be a 'field' for someone who wanted to study the process of experimentation rather than conducting the experiment itself. The important point here is that the field situation is naturally occurring: it is an episode in the ordinary, everyday, life of the people who are taking part in it.

The observer may come into this situation in one of four roles (Gold, 1958): complete participant; participant-as-observer; observer-as-participant; complete observer.

Definitions

There are various roles in fieldwork:

Complete participant is where the researcher is undercover. They are the only person who knows that their involvement in the situation is different from that of the people for whom it is everyday life. This is not necessarily the same as covert research: the fieldworker may be documenting their own life or workplace at the same time as they are carrying out their regular activities.

Participant-as-observer is where both researcher and researched know that observation is happening, but the researcher is also actively involved in the everyday life of the situation. This is probably the commonest role in field research.

Observer-as-participant is where the researcher uses a brief exposure to a situation to observe openly what is going on without any pretence of participating. If you are doing an interview on a ward, for example, this is also an opportunity to see something of its organisation and culture as activity goes on around you.

Complete observer is where the researcher has no direct interactional engagement with anyone in the situation they are studying. Examples might include eavesdropping on conversations in a hospital cafeteria or watching an operation on CCTV to examine the non-verbal communication between members of the surgical team.

These roles are not static, and the observer's involvement may shift between them from moment to moment during a session of fieldwork.

─────────────── **VIDEO SUPPORT** ───────────────

For a visual introduction to observational methods you can watch *Participant Observation and Structured Observation*. You can access the video by visiting this book's online resources: https://study.sagepub.com/dingwallandstaniland.

The important point here is to know which role you are playing at any particular moment. Why? Well, this is where the questions of reliability and validity that we discussed earlier come into play – and how observational research comes to be recognised as the gold standard for qualitative methods.

All social science research is influenced to some extent by the actions of the researchers who design a study and carry it out. Different methods try to deal with these influences in different ways. Some involve creating very strict instructions for how the research should be done – but even when you give telephone interviewers a script to follow, they still improvise. Psychological experiments put their subjects into artificial situations where they know they are being experimented on and try to work out what they are supposed to be doing. Qualitative methods just accept that researcher influences are unavoidable and try to identify them so that they can make explicit adjustments during the analysis phase. This is often discussed as *reflexivity*, where the researcher evaluates their own role in creating the data that they are reporting, either directly or indirectly.

CASE STUDY SCENARIO

Dingwall (1977 and Dingwall 2014) carried out two studies of health visitors, at the beginning and end of the 1970s. The first was for his PhD and the nurses he worked with assumed that he knew very little about their social world. As a result, they tended to treat him like a nursing student and explain their actions as they went along. He did not actually have to ask very many questions in the field. By the time of the second project, RD had published a book, papers in academic journals, and articles in professional magazines about the PhD research. Because relatively few people had ever done research on health visitors, his name had become quite familiar within their community. His expertise was taken for granted by the people that he worked with, so they did not think they needed to explain what they were doing. He had to devise strategies for getting them to talk about their work without appearing to be stupid or to have learned nothing from his previous research. Why would you waste time on someone who learned nothing? Why would you trust someone who was pretending to know less than they obviously did? Mostly, in fact, he explicitly used his expertise to talk about practice he had seen elsewhere and to ask why it was different here. Sometimes, he would imagine plausible alternative actions and ask why these might not be chosen. In contrast, Topsy Murray, his junior colleague, who had no previous exposure to health visitors, was able to collect the sort of data that RD had collected as a PhD student. By comparing data from the two projects and from the different observers at different career stages, RD and Topsy were able to construct a fuller understanding of health visitor practice and their own respective influences on the data they had collected. This allowed them to make stronger claims about both the reliability and the validity of the analyses that they developed. The second project was particularly well-resourced: it remains today one of the biggest qualitative studies ever carried out in the UK.

How can you check what you are seeing and hearing? One part of this is to compare your observations to the published literature. As we said earlier, this is why reading matters – and not just reading studies from nursing. In her study of quality assurance processes in a big hospital, KS read widely about similar processes in other large organisations and the ways in which they served purposes quite different from those that were the official rationale. This led her to recognise how a quality process that had no impact on everyday nursing care could still be successful because it enhanced the reputation of the hospital and attracted more recognition and funding, if the reports the hospital sent out externally said the right things. If the quality process had been considered only as a contribution to nursing standards, it would have been judged a failure and its other benefits would have been missed. We shall come back to this in Chapter 8, which focuses on documents, because they were central to this achievement.

The other check is to consider who the audience might be for the words and actions that you are observing. When you are doing observation, the people you are studying are mostly performing for each other. They may try to edit this to make a good impression on the observer, but it is hard to do that consistently.

For example, if you have ever been on a ward that is being visited by royalty, a politician or a celebrity, you will know how everyone is expected to put on a good show. Extra cleaners appear, fresh uniforms are issued, shifts are juggled to ensure attractive and pliable people are on duty. We sometimes call this a 'Potemkin village'.

Definition

Potemkin Village comes from the supposed efforts of Grigory Potemkin, who was the chief minister and lover of Catherine the Great, Empress of Russia, to create an appearance of the country's wealth and prosperity during a tour that she made in 1787. As she travelled down the Dnieper River, his men built fake villages on the banks and pretended to live in them. After she passed, the villages were dismantled, rushed downstream and rebuilt. Although modern scholarship suggests that this was actually a story invented by Potemkin's political enemies, the term has come to be applied to any temporary attempt to make a place or an organisation seem better than it actually is.

However, no organisation can keep this up for very long and everyday routines soon reassert themselves when the ceremonies are finished and the visitor has left. Observation goes through a similar process in a more limited way. Whatever people try to do in the first few hours to create a good impression is soon overtaken by the practicalities of getting through the work in ways that everyone is used to. This does not mean that the data from those first few hours are useless because it tells you how the people would like you to see them – and how they see you. Do they think you are there to judge them or to understand them?

CASE STUDY SCENARIO

Judging or understanding?

Despite my assurances that I was just observing everyday practice for research purposes, I was introduced to the doctors as 'a tutor from the school come to check up on us'. When asked whether I was observing doctors as well, I responded in the same frame of mind, that I liked to keep a keen eye on them. This however appeared to make no difference to practice in this instance, when the same doctor asked a patient to lie on his side and took a dressing off his back to examine a wound. The ward sister, who was pulling the curtains around the bed at the same time, turned and said to him, in front of the patient, 'You haven't washed your hands.' He did not respond and carried on talking to the patient. I noted however that he did not touch anything else and that he washed his hands before he left the bay. (Field notes: Staniland, 2008)

When you then start to ask people questions, those concerns are revived. They are likely to be looking to answer in ways that make them personally appear to be reasonable, rational and ethical and, in other respects, competent to do what they are doing. Social scientists call this *giving accounts* rather than *literal descriptions* of what they are thinking or feeling or what their motives were in acting as they have done (Dingwall, 1997).

Interviews only collect the accounts that are produced for the interviewer. Observation allows you to put these alongside the accounts that people produce for each other. How do you get to be regarded as a competent nurse by the people around you at some particular moment? Just what is it that you are saying and doing that leads them to that conclusion? Interviews take you away from that live moment. We are not implying that interviews are useless. Sometimes you do need quicker answers than observation can deliver. In many circumstances, a finding that is 80 per cent right and comes within a few weeks is more useful than a finding that is 95 per cent right and takes five years. One response has been to develop more rapid approaches to fieldwork such as Pink and Morgan (2013). Sometimes, you are interested in parts of people's lives that are difficult to access. If you want to know about sexual behaviour and the transmission of STIs, then you are likely to have to ask about it rather than observe it – although there have been (controversial) studies where the observer took up with sexual partners and wrote about the experience (Bolton, 1995). We shall come back to this in the next chapter and suggest some ways in which interviews can get closer to the action they are supposed to be capturing.

While we are encouraging you to be cautious about how you deal with what people say to you, this does not mean that you should not talk to them! We are discussing *participant* observation and, if you are going to participate, then of course you are going to talk to the people you are working with. These conversations sometimes take the form of *natural interviews*, where you ask people to explain their actions, their reasoning or their motives to you. If you go back to RD's description of his second health visitor study, you should be able to see that this is what he was doing when he compared the practice he was studying to observations or reports from other places. This case study is another example from KS:

CASE STUDY SCENARIO

At one point, I observed a cleaner who was busy wiping the cot sides of an occupied bed in one of the side bays. The patient had *Methicillin-resistant Staphylococcus aureus* (MRSA) and was being nursed in isolation. As I watched, the cleaner went from the cot sides to the bin outside the bay and carefully, using the same cloth, wiped that as well. I asked the sister if the ward had separate cleaners for MRSA-infected patients in bays. 'No,' she responded, 'cleaning is a problem, we are always short.' I asked how often these bays were cleaned and she did not know. She appeared not to have noticed the activities of the cleaner. (Staniland, 2008)

Natural interviews are embedded in the situation that you are studying, because you are asking questions as events are unfolding or very soon afterwards. They do not happen at a separate time and place. Although participant observers tend to emphasise the given nature of their data, their work often relies on material that they have solicited or provoked from participants. It is important that data collection, and analysis, acknowledge the difference between what is overheard or witnessed and what is generated by the direct intervention of the fieldworker. Occasionally, (although it can be a risky strategy for inexperienced researchers), a fieldworker may try to discover more about a setting by deliberately breaching one or more of its everyday conventions. The following, unpublished, example is taken from RD's work on child protection when he became interested in understanding how social workers stuck to professional standards when no-one was immediately watching what they were doing.

CASE STUDY SCENARIO

One particularly trusted informant was dealing with a pregnant teenager on her caseload and considering how to tell an absent and disengaged parent about her decision to give consent to an abortion without running the risk of prompting parental intervention. RD pointed out that she had the option of writing such a letter, placing a copy on the file and destroying the original, blaming non-receipt on the postal service if subsequently challenged by the parent.

He used her, negative, reaction to this suggestion as a means of exploring her sense of professionally or organisationally-correct behaviour and subsequently used the episode in natural interviews with other social workers to determine whether the temptation and rejection would be recognisable to them. KS's behaviour when the doctor ignored the ward sister's reprimand for not washing his hands is similar.

CRITICAL THINKING EXERCISE

Ethics as they happen

Why do you think KS did not intervene when the doctor ignored the ward sister's comment? When we wrote about ethics in Chapter 5, we discussed the responsibility of nurses to protect patients from harm and the difference that this might make when they were doing fieldwork. Should KS have spoken out as well?

This is a good example of the sort of ethical decision that you might have to make in the moment, much as RD made his social worker take. This does not get covered by ethics review processes and approvals. We would justify KS's choice by noting that the sister did not follow up on her comment and insist that the doctor washed his hands. This is different from the example we gave earlier of seeing a student or an assistant doing something risky. An experienced nurse had decided not to go on challenging the doctor's actions on this occasion. This told KS something about how the sister assessed risk, that the actions were not ideal but not 'really' dangerous, and about the ways in which even senior nurses on this ward deferred to doctors. KS did not think that she should disrupt the scene she was observing by going beyond what the sister thought was appropriate. The longer-term interests of the research outweighed a theoretical risk to the patient that did not seem greatly to concern any of the people she was observing.

Do you agree with our reasoning here?
(In your rationale, try to also bear in mind your own professional code of practice. As a nurse, you are also an advocate for patients. The risk of biasing research results has to be balanced against complying with a professional code).

IN THE FIELD

This section looks at three practical issues that people often feel anxious about when they first go into the field. Remember there is nothing magic about doing participant observation. This is one classic list of fieldwork skills: 'active looking, improving memory, informal interviewing, writing detailed field notes, and perhaps most importantly, patience' (DeWalt and DeWalt, 2010: x). These are skills that you use all the time in your everyday life – and your professional practice. Fieldwork just asks you to use them in a more self-conscious fashion so you can polish them to a higher level.

Of course, now you have improved these skills, you can take that learning back into other contexts. It will, for example, help you to listen more closely to your patients or to think more carefully about how they will respond to the way you talk to them. There are, though, a few specific challenges that we should look at.

VIDEO SUPPORT

You may wish to watch *What to Observe in Participant Observation* before you study this section. You can access the video by visiting this book's online resources: https://study.sagepub.com/dingwallandstaniland.

GAINING ACCESS

Access for field research needs to be negotiated at two levels. First, you are likely to need the permission of senior people in the research setting you want to study. Your course probably has a protocol about this and your supervisor should guide you through that. Even if you just want to study other students, your university is likely to have policies that are intended to ensure that their goodwill is not abused. The people at this level who are giving the approval are usually described as the *gatekeepers* for your research. You will need to think about how to write a description of what you want to do that shows them you are serious and that it is worth allowing you to use their organisation's time and resources on your project. You should revisit Chapter 3 when you are doing this. You will probably not need to go into as much detail as your course or ethics review committee would require, but you must persuade them that you know what you are doing – and that *it is in their interest to co-operate*. This last phrase is important. This is not about you telling them what you want to do, but you explaining that what you want to do is potentially useful for them, or for people like them. This also helps you with the steps required for the research. When we discuss writing up, we shall explain more about the 'imagined reader'. Right now, let's just say that you should write a draft and then use your imagination to put yourself in the place of the person you are trying to persuade. Why would they let you loose in one of their wards or clinics?

However, there is a lot more to access than getting a sign-off from the director of nursing services or whoever; you also have to establish a relationship with the people you are actually studying! This is the second level of negotiation. The boss may have agreed, but this does not guarantee that anyone else will go along with it.

CASE STUDY SCENARIO

During his child protection research, RD spent some time in the A&E department of a large, prestigious teaching hospital. Although he had the agreement of the consultants to carry out fieldwork, the junior doctors and nurses did not feel they had been adequately consulted. They were also very sceptical about the value of qualitative research. As a result, RD encountered quite a lot of hostility and lack of co-operation. On one occasion, for example, he was asked, quite inappropriately, to monitor an emotionally distressed patient, only to discover that all the professional staff had retreated to the ward office to drink tea and gossip. The premature end of the fieldwork came about when the junior doctors realised that they had been observed in unofficial adjustments of their shifts on the night of the hospital ball. Staff who were on duty were leaving to spend time at the ball, while others ducked in from the ball to cover their absence. A deputation to the consultants resulted in RD's access being withdrawn.

You are not likely to have such a bad time, but you should understand that these things happen even to experienced researchers!

Many student projects are carried out in the places where they are currently working. This can present some challenges in terms of separating a work role from a research role, which we will look at when we discuss note-taking. Suppose, though, that you do decide to do your project in a place where people do not know you. What do you do when you meet the people you are going to study?

One way to approach this is to use the skills that you are developing by learning about qualitative research. Meeting the people you are going to study is one of a class of situations that we might call *first days* – we nearly wrote 'first dates'. All through your life, there are things you have done for the first time. The first day at school, a first day at university, first day in practice – or first meeting with a potential romantic partner. How did you act on those occasions? What did you do to smooth your path and learn how to fit in? Typically, people hold back a little from expressing their own views or initiating actions. They do more listening and watching to see how other people are acting. When they do talk or act, they do this in a tentative fashion, carefully monitoring the reactions of those around them. They try to spot who might be particularly supportive to a newbie. You have often been in that situation and observed others in that situation. When a new patient comes onto your ward or into your clinic, you can see the difference in their behaviour from those who are familiar and experienced.

When you are doing participant observation, first days are actually the source of some of the most valuable data. After a while, you get used to the setting and you take all sorts of things for granted that are really uncertain in those initial encounters. The first day – the things you get right and the things you get wrong – makes that setting more transparent than usual. Be sure to write all this down in the ways we will discuss shortly.

SAMPLING: BEING IN THE RIGHT PLACE (AT THE RIGHT TIME)

One of the things that new observational researchers often ask us is: what do I actually do? How do I organise my observation time? The most efficient way of doing this is *shadowing*. In health care settings, this usually takes one of three forms:

- *Person shadowing* is where the fieldworker is attached to a specific individual, tracking them through their routine work for an agreed period of time. Very often this is something that comes out of a first day experience, where someone decides to sponsor the newbie and show them around. This needs to be handled with some caution because you will normally want to do the same with other people, possibly from different grades in the setting, and you should be sure that your first choice does not cut you off from others.
- *Place shadowing* is where the fieldworker picks a particular location and watches what happens there. RD's study of the A&E department was intended to be an example of this. His intention was to observe how work and information flows were co-ordinated between different groups of professional and non-professional staff. From this he expected to work out how decisions were made about whether children's injuries were accidental or non-accidental.
- *Patient shadowing* may have elements of place shadowing if the patient is spending most of their time in a bed. However, it is worth distinguishing because the observer is following a patient through their experience of a medical organisation. This may involve meeting a number of different staff in different locations. It might involve, for example, going from a clinic to a scanning or X-ray suite and then onwards to another clinic to assess the results.

When planning shadowing, do not forget that you might also want to sample a field site by *time*. Many health care organisations work quite differently at nights and weekends. People's jobs change. Different kinds of case are dealt with. Some rules and practices are relaxed. Quite a few expansions of nursing roles have come about because researchers asked why it was acceptable for a nurse to give a drug, or perform a task usually done by a doctor, at 03:00 hrs on Sunday morning but not at 15:00 hrs on a Wednesday afternoon.

WRITING FIELD NOTES

Definition

Field notes are a kind of evidence on which inquirers base claims about meaning and understanding. However, there is no standard definition of field notes, their form, or content. Some fieldworkers define field notes as raw data or material – notes made in the field based on observations and conversations, rough diagrams and charts, lists of terms, and so on. These notes can contain descriptions of episodes and events, scene depictions, and sketches. They may also contain reflections and interpretations of members' meanings, points of view, and so on. Others contrast field notes with data, defining field notes more along the lines of daily entries made in a field journal to record thoughts, impressions, initial ideas, working hypotheses, issues to pursue, and so on. For some, field notes include all those things collected in the course of fieldwork – the fieldwork journal, transcripts of conversations and interviews, photographs, audiotapes and videotapes, copies of documents and artefacts. Others exclude some of these as not

> belonging to field notes proper. This wide variation in defining field notes is attributable to the fact that these kinds of notes are very much prepared for an audience of one – the fieldworker – and thus are individualistic and personal and reflective of the unique ways individual fieldworkers conduct fieldwork. (Schwandt, 2015:117)

Field notes are the primary source of evidence for most observational studies. While it is possible that they will eventually be superseded by bodycams, as we discuss later, this is not likely to happen rapidly: there may still be many situations where note-taking remains important. How do you take notes? What do you take notes about? Neither of these questions has a right answer, it depends upon the context.

In an ideal situation, you can carry a notebook (the most useful kind are those that used to be sold to journalists with a spiral wire binding that can flip over rapidly to give you a fresh page. These are compact and will generally fit into a pocket or a handbag.) Make sure that the beginning of each session of observation has a note of the time and place and that the notebook is clearly marked to identify it in case you lose it. You can then hover on the edge of the interactions you are observing and make notes as things are going on. Very few people can do this in shorthand nowadays so you will probably develop your own codes or abbreviations for recording words and actions. You make the initial note visibly and in real time. This is mostly what we did in our own studies. Today, you could probably do the same with a stylus and an electronic notepad, but the old technology does not have the same risks of flat batteries and software failures.

———————————————— VIDEO SUPPORT ————————————————

The short video *How to Write an Effective Field Note* offers tips on writing field notes. You can access the video by visiting this book's online resources: https://study.sage-pub.com/dingwallandstaniland.

However, there are occasions on which this is not possible.

CASE STUDY SCENARIO

When RD was observing informal pub lunches supposed to promote good relations between social workers and health visitors, for example, he just scribbled key words on a beer mat or slipped off to the toilet to make slightly longer notes. When he studied a genetics laboratory, he would sometimes edge round the back of the cupboards or refrigerators to be less visible, especially if one member of the lab had just been critical of another's practice.

In a study of student 'lad culture', supervised by RD, the researcher dictated brief notes into her mobile phone while observing interactions between students. So many people were using their phones in these bars and clubs that this method was less obtrusive than sitting with a notebook and pen. If you are observing in your own workplace, you may also find it difficult to make notes visibly around your colleagues. You could think of carrying a second, smaller, notebook that you can use quickly to note things that your colleagues might feel threatened by if they saw you writing in the main notebook.

These immediate jottings are written in the field at the time, or as near to the event as possible. They are intended to help you remember what you saw and heard so that you can reconstruct it more accurately later. You should treat them as highly personal and confidential documents. They are likely to contain material that is very sensitive. Some of it might be damaging to the people who have allowed you to observe them and to the organisations where they work. Remember that KS initially thought that the quality assurance process she observed was a serious waste of time and money. It was only when she began to review her notes that she realised the ways in which it had actually been a success for the hospital. By the time data are published, they have been through an intense editing process that is intended to disguise its sources, in ways that do not compromise the analytic points. However, data do not begin like that.

When you leave the field site at the end of a session of observation, your work is only half done. This is one of the things that makes fieldwork such an intense experience. Your next task is to take your scribblings and turn them into the documents that you will actually use in your analysis. These are the field notes proper, where you use your jottings to help you reconstruct an accurate, detailed and coherent description of exactly what you saw and what you heard. This reconstruction should also make it clear where the participants appeared to be reacting to your presence or where they did something that you had prompted. Were they talking to each other or responding to a question you had asked? Did they imply that some procedure was being done 'by the book' only because you were watching? This process should happen as soon as possible after the period of observation. In a perfect world, you would probably do it immediately, but we all have other things going on in our lives. Just don't leave it more than a day or two at the most. Plan this time into your fieldwork schedule. Observe for half days or half shifts or half weeks so you build in opportunities to transcribe your jottings.

Do not try to summarise or interpret in these notes. Imagine you are the Recording Angel, tasked to log, impartially and impassively, the events, actions and achievements of each individual human life to determine their eternal fate. These notes should use real names, repeat actual words so far as possible and specify dates, times and places. Ask yourself: 'If I had to go to court and answer questions from a lawyer, would these notes be sufficiently detailed for my answers to be credible?' Again, we must stress the sensitivity of this material. You should not share it with anyone other than your immediate supervisor or, possibly, an examiner. Once the project is finished, you must consider whether to destroy these notes, and the jottings that preceded them, or archive them securely – your supervisor should be able to advise you about this, in line with university policies. Remember, though, that personal responsibility for the security of field data is part of the great tradition of qualitative research. It means as much to social scientists as patient confidentiality does to a truly professional nurse.

Key Point

At the same time as producing field notes, many researchers find it helpful to be writing a separate document that contains their reflections and preliminary thoughts on analysis. This is where you can record your thoughts about what the data mean and how they might be similar to, or different from, other studies that you have read. (You may already have experience of this if you think back to the reflections you wrote as a student.) You will come back to this when you are analysing the data because it is likely to contain many of the first traces of the themes that you are identifying.

What are you going to take notes about? Reed (1995:48) gives an example of a common starting problem. Following two hours of fieldwork on an elderly care ward, her 'sheets of paper were as blank as they had been at the beginning of the session'.

When she went over her experience with her supervisor, however, the discussion progress from 'nothing interesting had happened' to 'in the space of two hours nurses had got 24 patients out of bed, toileted, washed and dressed them and given them their medications and breakfasts'. What has happened here? Essentially, Reed had not managed to accomplish the difficult task of treating a field site with which she was very familiar as 'anthropologically strange'. What do we mean by this?

Observational research began with people going to places that were intrinsically strange. Anthropologists worked with the indigenous peoples of Africa, Australasia and the Americas. Sociologists left their middle-class homes and universities to study poor, working-class and minority people where they lived and worked. Today, the observers are more diverse – but so are the settings. When we are studying a social world that is very familiar to us, we have to work quite hard to imagine how it looks to someone who is meeting it for the first time. This is why we used the metaphor of the Recording Angel just now. Other writers have suggested you could think of yourself as a Martian studying the peoples of Planet Earth.

This is why it has taken us a long time to get to the practical bits of this book. The key to knowing what to write in your jottings and field notes is the quality of your reading and your research question. What do you need to record to answer that? It is important not to overdo this. One of the strengths of fieldwork is the ability to discover new questions or unexpected insights. But you must have somewhere to start from, a 'foreshadowed problem'. If you are just hanging out and waiting for inspiration to strike, you will waste a lot of time. This may be part of the legend of fieldwork, but it is not efficient. Remember when we introduced Zeno the Stoic. His outstretched hand represented your willingness to engage with the world. The gradual closing of his hand represented your decisions about what you were going to select from the possibilities that the world offered you.

CASE STUDY SCENARIO

Here is one example from our own experience. Some years ago, RD was invited to do some brief fieldwork in a university genetics research laboratory. There is a tradition of similar studies in the sociology of science, but this was a very open invitation: come and see what you can find. While this is not the kind of invitation that you are likely to get, it actually presents an experienced field-worker with the same problem: 'I have just been asked to come without a specific research question, so what should I take notes about?'

RD drew a map of the lab, collected some biographies from the PhD students, postdocs and technicians, and looked over people's shoulders as they did some experiments. One postdoc, for example, showed him a Petri dish where the introduction of an antibiotic had selectively eliminated various bacterial colonies. It proved the point he had been trying to establish – but it was not neat enough to photograph for publication. If he were working in an industrial lab, he would move on to the next experiment. Since he wanted to publish rather than develop a product, he planned to redo the experiment to get a more elegant result. Previous studies had commented on the degree to which science rested on a set of craft skills that were not much discussed among scientists. This interaction suggested that there might also be an aesthetic dimension to science and pointed to potentially interesting ways in which university and industry practice might differ.

RD also noticed that different lab members wore different styles of lab coat, and started to make systematic notes of who wore what when. One condition for his access had been that the lab's principal investigator would be able to read his field notes, towards the possibility of a joint publication. She was puzzled by this focus on something so trivial. In fact, as RD explained, this was not, from his point of view, a trivial observation. He was referring back to research from the 1950s by Julius Roth (1957) in a hospital for TB patients. Roth noticed that protective clothing was a symbolic marker of status boundaries. The higher the status of the person, the less likely they were to wear masks or gowns: the bacillus would not dare to travel on a doctor's clothing but might do on a ward cleaner's.

There is a useful example of this which took place during the 2020 pandemic involving the Vice President of America, Mike Pence, not wearing a mask! You can read the BBC News article on this on the website at https://study.sagepub.com/dingwallandstaniland. The British Prime Minister, Boris Johnson, also ostentatiously shook hands with patients in a general hospital at the beginning of the pandemic episode in the UK – you can watch a YouTube video of the incident on the book's website.

Anyone could see the hierarchy of workers just by looking at what they wore on the wards. RD had been influenced by this finding during his PhD research on health visitors in the early 1970s. Their employer had just stopped requiring them to wear a uniform, giving them vouchers to buy 'civilian' clothing instead. However, these vouchers could only be exchanged at rather conservative department stores, so the employer still controlled the 'professional' image presented by its staff.

When RD went into the unfamiliar setting of the laboratory and was inducted into its health and safety requirements for standard protective clothing, he was immediately alert to the possibility that there might be some organisational significance to the different styles of lab coat that were actually being worn. Because he knew the principal investigator would read the field notes, he had also left out the lab gossip he had picked up about a postdoc who had recently been reprimanded for persistent breaches of the clothing requirements.

This experience underlines several earlier points:

- RD was drawing on his background reading and previous research to identify something that might be important in the field site. He had foreshadowed a possible line of inquiry. Fieldwork is not an aimless process.
- At the same time, he was open to the specific significance that the choice of lab coats might have in this context. Wearing the right clothing in the right way demonstrated a 'correct' understanding of the lab's practices. This was different from Roth's observations about infection risk and status, although it had some association with his own previous work on how health visitors demonstrated their professionalism.
- RD had also made a quick ethical decision to omit certain details where he could not guarantee the confidentiality of his observations. The material seen by his host was only what would have been available to her in the open, everyday, interactions in the lab. RD might have identified other issues in those interactions, as with the bacterial culture that was not elegant enough, but he had respected the sensitivity of the things other lab members said in less public spaces.

AUDIO AND VIDEO RECORDING

The big disadvantage about taking field notes by hand is that you cannot avoid losing potentially important information. No one can write fast enough to capture all the details of talk. You cannot take another look at a site if you think you might have missed something relevant in the people's actions or their environment. Since the 1960s, however, the introduction of increasingly lightweight and compact audio and video recorders has made it possible to review and replay talk and actions almost indefinitely. These data can also be shared with colleagues and analyses refined in workshops that constrain the subjectivity of any one researcher.

This technology has opened up whole new areas of research and analysis (see Parry et al., 2016). In turn, these have allowed us to identify new kinds of intervention to achieve practical changes in many settings, particularly in health care. Recording technologies are becoming so portable that researchers are beginning to experiment with bodycams that record every moment of their day. This is called *lifelogging*. Social science and health care ethics regulators have been hostile to this development, but computer science ethics committees have been more liberal in their approach. As people gain more familiarity with the idea, it is likely that bodycams will be used more in research. They might be worn by fieldworkers or by participants themselves, with the fieldworker collecting them in at the end of an agreed session or, more likely, recording remotely over a wireless connection.

Before you rush to embrace such technologies, though, you should think carefully about whether they are really appropriate ways of investigating the questions you are interested in. We have already mentioned the challenge of getting past ethics regulators. Even if you could achieve that, there are three issues you need to think about. First, recording yields masses of data that need a lot of time to work through, transcribe and analyse. Second, recording only captures what happens to be within range at the time – current devices cannot match the 360° view and the selective attention of a human observer. Third, it can be difficult to edit into a form suitable for publication, communicating the important details but adequately disguising the participants. For these reasons, we think that traditional human observation will continue to be important for the foreseeable future. Remember what we said about getting something 80 per cent right in a reasonable time and at a reasonable cost possibly being more useful than being 95 per cent right as a result of a longer and more expensive project.

There are two particular areas where audio and video recording have made a big impact: the study of interactions between health professionals and their patients or clients; and the study of situations where close collaborative working is important, like operating theatres. This research draws on two linked approaches in social science called *ethnomethodology* and, as we describe later, *conversation* (or sometimes *discourse*) *analysis*.

> **Definition**
>
> **Ethnomethodology** is a term coined by the American sociologist, Harold Garfinkel, to describe investigation of the ways (methods) that ordinary people (ethnos) make their world seem orderly and coherent through their everyday interactions.

─────────────────────────── **VIDEO SUPPORT** ───────────────────────────

You can access a video explaining *Ethnomethodology* by visiting this book's online resources: https://study.sagepub.com/dingwallandstaniland.

While you may not have an opportunity to do research of this kind, its impact on studies of patient–professional communication and on the co-ordination of medical and surgical teamwork means that it is important to be aware of what it has to offer.

In the early 1950s, Garfinkel worked on a project studying how US jurors made decisions in criminal trials (vom Lehn, 2016). Their jury room discussions were recorded with the heavy-duty equipment of the time. When he listened to the recordings, Garfinkel realised that the jurors were discussing issues of evidence, truth and falsity in ways that paralleled similar discussions among scientists and scholars. Everyone was concerned with these issues in their own way. However, while philosophers and social scientists were studying their own discussions, no one at the time was very interested in investigating how such matters were dealt with by ordinary people. His efforts to stimulate work on this topic inspired a small but increasingly influential line of research. One example is Lorenza Mondada's (2014) study of collaboration during surgical operations.

Mondada had access to about 25 hours of video recordings of laparoscopic and open surgery, made by the surgeons for their own use. This particular paper focuses on an open operation for an inguinal hernia and the ways in which the surgeon and his assistant co-ordinate the use of their hands. If you just listen to the verbal directions given by the surgeon, they are a series of very short, direct instructions. Mondada shows that these instructions only make sense when they are placed into the context of actions with the surgical instruments and the changing character of the tissues being dissected. They are complemented by non-verbal directions – pointing with an instrument or pushing a tissue towards the assistant to pick up and grasp with their tools – and by assistants apparently intuitively acting on their own initiative. The assistant shows that they understand what they are supposed to be doing without needing to be told. This is not a matter of telepathy. The surgeon and the assistant are both orienting to an unfolding sequence of actions that ultimately produce the outcome for the patient. The sequence is created jointly and, in the moment, although obviously both are bringing their 'professional vision' (Goodwin 1994), the result of previous training and experiences, to this particular operation.

What might this mean for practice? Like Garfinkel's jurors, the surgeon and the assistant were working to create an appearance of orderliness. For the jurors, their findings had to be acceptable as rational outcomes of the material presented in the trial. For the surgical team, the outcome of the operation was, ideally, a smooth technical process where any problems or uncertainties were resolved along the way. However, the apparent order of the operation was not the result of following a script but of skilled improvisation, where the team members could draw on their experience and signal their moves to each other as they were required.

——————————————— FREEING OUR IMAGINATION ———————————————

You might go on from this, for example, to be interested in how well such co-ordination works among people who do not share experiences or have not previously worked together. If a surgeon, an anaesthetist and a theatre nurse meet for the first time at the beginning of a list, will they be able to work in the way that Mondada and others have described?

Studying a few minutes of one operation in very great detail provokes a very big question for patient safety.

Conversation analysis is closely related to ethnomethodology.

Definition

Conversation analysis is a specific application of ethnomethodology to identify and describe the methods that people use to produce and interpret social interaction. It involves the detailed study of practices such as greetings, giving directions or telling stories.

Both approaches share a concern to understand the way in which the apparent orderliness of the world is created by what people do – rather than being 'out-there' and separate from them. The world is *improvised* rather than *scripted*. Conversation analysis begins from an observation that social scientists first made in the 18th century, that the meaning of an action was not identifiable from the intentions of its producer but from the response of those who received or observed it. Because humans are not telepathic, the only evidence that we have about intentions comes from what we can see and hear. We make inferences from this as a basis for our responses. As with Mondada's surgeons, we also use our previous knowledge and experiences to make those inferences but each occasion is potentially new and different. If the person who produced the action does not like our responses, they can, of course, try to *correct* or *repair* our misunderstanding. We can represent this as a three-turn structure that is the basis of all interactions (see Figure 6.1).

Turn Speaker	Turn Hearer
1 Statement, question etc.	
	2 Response
3 Correction, repair etc. *or* Next statement, question etc.	

Figure 6.1   Three-turn structure of interactions

In practice, of course, things are a lot more complicated than that, as we have discovered since we were able to record and replay interactions in a way that earlier social scientists could not.

This approach is called *conversation* analysis because the initial research was done, using the technology of the time, on telephone calls between friends in the Los Angeles area. In practice, it has been used very widely in health care settings to understand the interactions between professionals and their clients or patients. These include studies of doctors, pharmacists, nurses and physiotherapists, as well as related workers like call handlers dealing with emergency services. This work has fed into practice in areas like advice-giving, delivering bad news, responding to emergency calls and engaging patients in exercise treatments. Some useful practical resources were developed for the

---
VIDEO SUPPORT

Stokoe and Marlow provide another excellent visual introduction to conversational analysis in *Conversation Analysis: CARM Training*. You can access the video by visiting the book's online resources: https://study.sagepub.com/dingwallandstaniland. Another video, focusing on interaction analysis, can also be viewed by visiting the online resources: Rivas, *An Introduction to Interaction Analysis.*

COVID-19 pandemic, for example. These included advice on communication when wearing face masks and on breaking bad news over the telephone: www.realtalktraining.co.uk/posts (accessed 10/05/20).

One example of the way conversation analysis has changed thinking relates to the issue of power in medical consultations. In the past, many participant observers thought that doctor–patient and similar interactions were a display of power, where professionals subordinated, or even oppressed, service users and their concerns. They reached this conclusion largely by noting that professionals seemed to ask a lot of questions and, through these, to determine what was talked about during a consultation. This led to many proposals for training professionals to step back, to respond to questions from patients, and to share decision making. However, looking at studies from audio and video recordings of consultations since the 1970s, Alison Pilnick and Robert Dingwall (2011) found little or no evidence of actual changes in practice. Communication skills training in professional education seemed to have had no identifiable impact. They looked again at the evidence and argued that what was called 'power' actually reflected an inescapable inequality in knowledge. People consulted health professionals because they knew stuff that ordinary men and women did not. Many patients were very puzzled by the attempt to deny this and share decisions about diagnosis and treatment. Professionals asked a lot of questions simply because they needed to clarify the presenting problem and patients seemed to expect this. Similarly, where the professionals tried to withhold definite answers on diagnosis, prognosis and treatment options, the patients tried either to extract these or to find ways of inferring what the professionals were thinking. If we go back to Figure 6.1, patients would use their second position to try to force an expansion of whatever the professional had said in the first turn. This work is still controversial because many social scientists, and some health professionals, are attracted by the analysis of professional dominance for other reasons. However, it is an argument that can only happen because of the ability to listen closely and repeatedly to what is being said in an interaction.

CHAPTER SUMMARY POINTS

This chapter has considered some of the practical aspects of observing people. It has described the different roles that observers may take when studying the social processes involved in modern health care and identified some strengths and weaknesses of observational research. It has recognised field notes as a foundation of using observational research as data and identified the technological aids of audio and video recording to replay and review observations in different ways. Observational data are particularly valuable when:

- The nature of the research is focused on a what or how question.
- Little is known about the behaviour of people in any one setting.
- The research objective is to understand a site in a comprehensive and detailed way.
- The research objective is to understand some topic in its natural setting.
- Asking people about what they do is likely to elicit answers that are very different from their actual behaviour.

When implementing any intervention in a natural setting, observational data helps researchers to evaluate whether that intervention has been faithfully transferred across settings and to identify when the implementation has become stable and secure:

- Immersion and prolonged involvement in a setting can lead to the development of rapport and foster free and open speaking with members.
- Observation fosters an in-depth and rich understanding of a phenomenon, situation and/or setting and the behaviour of the participants in that setting.
- Observation is an essential part of gaining an understanding of natural settings and their members' ways of seeing.
- Observation provides a foundation for the development of more general theory and for hypotheses about how this might be tested by means of natural or artificial experiments.
- Observational data is a way to improve clinical skills – learning how to see things you would not otherwise have noticed.

Or for a fuller explanation of observation in research, see www.qualres.org/HomeObse-3594.html (accessed 27/2/20).

FURTHER READING

This chapter has cited a number of helpful sources for further reading about observational methods in general. Although we are not specifically dealing with qualitative research in low- and middle-income countries, you may be interested to look at the application of qualitative methods in a study of a South African hospital. This study is a particularly nice example of the integration of analyses from observations, interviews, documents and artefacts, which will be the theme of the next three chapters.

Hull, E. (2017) *Contingent Citizens: Professional Aspiration in a South African Hospital.* London: Bloomsbury.

If you want to know more about conversation analysis and ethnomethodology, there are a number of textbooks at a more advanced level. Two we particularly recommend are:

vom Lehn, D. (2016) *Harold Garfinkel: The Creation and Development of Ethnomethodology.* Abingdon: Routledge.

Garcia, A.C. (2013) *An Introduction to Interaction: Understanding Talk in Formal and Informal Settings.* London: Bloomsbury.

A more popular account of conversation analysis is

Stokoe, E. (2018) *Talk: The Science of of Conversation.* London: Robinson.

Some further examples of the use of these approaches in health care are:

Bloch, S. and Leydon, G. (2019) 'Conversation analysis and telephone helplines for health and illness: a narrative review', *Research on Language and Social Interaction*, 52(3): 193–211. Available at https://doi.org/10.1080/08351813.2019.1631035 (accessed 27/2/20).

Pecanac, K.E. (2018) 'Combining conversation analysis and event sequencing to study health communication', *Research in Nursing & Health*, 41(3): 312–19. Available at https://doi.org/10.1002/nur.21863 (accessed 27/2/20).

Sbaih, L.C. (2002) 'Meanings of immediate: the practical use of the Patient's Charter in the accident and emergency department', *Social Science and Medicine*, 54(9): 1345–55. Available at https://doi.org/10.1016/s0277-9536(01)00100-9 (accessed 27/2/20).

7

Interviewing People

> ## Learning Outcomes
>
> At the end of this chapter you will be able to:
>
> - Define and identify how to use a qualitative interview
> - Classify different types of qualitative interview
> - Identify how to prepare and categorise appropriate questions for a qualitative interview
> - Recognise the importance of designing an interview agenda and of sampling in qualitative interviews
> - Discuss the advantages and limitations of qualitative interviewing

In Chapter 6, we explained why participant observation, or hanging out, was considered to be the gold standard for qualitative research. However, most qualitative studies today rely more heavily on interviews, or asking questions. These are not the natural interviews that we discussed in the context of participant observation. They are set-piece discussions where the researcher and their informant meet for an agreed period of time to talk about some particular topic or set of topics.

Interview studies are more common because they are usually quicker and cheaper and can often be sub-contracted to students or research assistants. Sometimes they are the only way to find out about events that are difficult to observe, because they have already taken place, because they are uncommon, or because they tend to happen in private spaces. If you want to know about domestic violence, for example, this may be difficult to observe, even if you can get agreement to install recording equipment in someone's home. A less creditable reason for the growth in interview studies is their easier passage through research ethics committees: they are thought to be more controllable than observational studies, where risks are harder to assess in advance.

By this stage in your life, you will almost certainly have had extensive experience of being interviewed. Two leading qualitative researchers, Paul Atkinson and David Silverman (1997), have suggested that we live in an 'interview society', where most people are well used to being interviewed and talking about their lives and thoughts. You have probably been interviewed at school, at the entrance to your nursing course and for any jobs that you may have been shortlisted for. You may have taken place in market research interviews or focus groups. You may even have been stopped in the street for a 'vox pop' for radio or television. If you look at old cinema newsreels or early TV broadcasts, you can see how much people's behaviour has changed since the early 1950s. When someone puts a microphone under our nose, we now know exactly how to respond, with a fluent and focused sound bite.

———————— FREEING OUR IMAGINATION ————————

A widely-circulated sound bite

A short clip that you can access by visiting this book's online resources (https://study.sagepub.com/dingwallandstaniland) illustrates the fluency with which ordinary people can respond to media interviews in the street.

You may also have had experience of doing interviewing. It would be unusual as a nurse if you have not been involved in collecting information from patients who are being admitted to a ward or clinic. Perhaps you have been responsible for recruiting casual workers in a service industry like a bar or a café. Many school projects in subjects like geography involve interviewing people, although you may have been too shy to approach strangers and just sat on a park bench and made up the answers!

SELF-ASSESSMENT ACTIVITY

Take a few moments to make some notes about what you have learned from interviewing and being interviewed.
   The introduction here might suggest at least two points:

- You have had some practice in constructing stories about yourself and your ideas when people ask you to tell them.
- It can be difficult to know what you have found from an interview.

You can probably think of a few more.

In the last chapter, we suggested that thinking about participant observation would help you with professional practice. In the same way, thinking about how to ask questions *and listen to the responses* can be transferred to your interactions with patients, carers and colleagues. There is nothing magic about interviewing: it is an everyday skill that researchers have thought hard about, reflected on and tried to refine.

WHAT IS A QUALITATIVE INTERVIEW?

We think the best description of a qualitative interview is that it is a *'conversation with a purpose'* (Burgess, 1984: 102 our italics). What do we mean by this?

First, qualitative interviews do not have a fixed structure and wording, in the way that survey questionnaires mostly do. A survey may be carried out face to face by an interviewer, although the cost of doing this on a large scale means that it is now more commonly done by telephone, post or online. Whether a human interviewer is involved or not, the survey, in principle, asks everyone exactly the same questions in the same order with the same wording and the same options for answering. The answers to questions in survey interviews are normally entered directly onto paper or electronic devices with a built-in coding scheme that generates quantitative data. This can be summarised in tables or fed into statistical calculations to look for patterns in the responses. In practice, there may be some minor variations, if the answers to certain questions mean that others are dropped or included, creating different pathways through the interview. Sometimes there are also a few free-text questions where the interviewer writes down the *respondent*'s own words rather than ticking a box.

Qualitative interviews, on the other hand, roam more freely so that topics are dealt with as they arise, and the *informant's* responses are discussed to establish what they are intending to communicate. Informants are encouraged to 'speak in their own voice and express their own thoughts and feelings' (Berg, 2007: 96; see also Lune and Berg, 2017: 105–165). These interviews may be recorded by hand, in much the same way as we described for field notes, although audio devices are often used; they may also occasionally be videoed. The data are produced in the free text of notes or transcripts, from which extracts are quoted in the final report.

Although qualitative researchers try to make their interviews feel like conversations, it is important not to forget the second part of Burgess's description: they have a *purpose*, they are not random chats. This means that they require planning to create an underlying structure and logic that will allow relevant data to be collected. This structure may be less visible and more flexible than that of a survey questionnaire, but it is just as necessary. It usually takes the form of an *agenda*, where the interviewer lists the information they hope to obtain and possibly suggests some question wording as a prompt to themselves. The order of topics may change, and new ones may be added as the interview unfolds. The interviewer may learn from their informant how they can better phrase their questions. At some points, the informant may take over and impose their concerns. However, nobody's time should be wasted on an interview that does not collect the information required by the study.

It is important not to exaggerate the differences between these types of interview or to suggest that one is better than the other. The vital thing is to know which one you should be doing at the time. Do you need to answer questions that come in a quantitative form – how much, how many, how often? Or are you asking questions about processes – how come this happened, how does this work, why was this the outcome of that action? Qualitative and quantitative interviews are different solutions to the problem of *equivalence*. This is the challenge of knowing when one person's answers to a question are similar to another's. Have they actually understood the question in the same way? Are we justified in putting them in the same category, whether or not we intend to count the numbers in that category? Interviews that are structured by a survey or a questionnaire assume that fixed sequences and question wording will produce comparable answers. The person who is providing the information is merely required to *respond*. This assumption is justifiable for certain kinds of data whose character is so widely understood that we can call it *factual* – although, as we shall see in the next chapter, this may not be an easy assumption to make.

Interviews that are structured by an agenda assume that flexible sequences and question designs by a skilled researcher are needed to get behind the initial descriptions provided to them by people who are trying to *inform* them about their place in the world. The comparability is produced by digging into what people *mean* rather than what they *say*. The danger, of course, is that the comparability is then actually produced by the interviewer rather than by their informant – social scientists sometimes call this *co-construction*. Can you be sure that your categories come from your informants rather than from your own starting assumptions?

Do not worry if you find this a bit difficult to grasp. We shall come back to all of these topics in the course of the chapter. They will be explained in more detail and we will suggest practical ways in which you can manage the problems that we have just identified.

Key Point

Qualitative researchers tend to describe the people who they interview as 'informants' or 'participants' rather than 'respondents' or 'interviewees'. This stresses the active role that they are thought to play in the research – they do not just respond to a researcher's questioning, but they inform the researcher about themselves and their experiences.

VIDEO SUPPORT

How to Plan and Conduct Interviews in a Research Project offers tips to help you plan and conduct a qualitative interview. You can access the video by visiting this book's online resources: https://study.sagepub.com/dingwallandstaniland.

WHEN SHOULD YOU USE QUALITATIVE INTERVIEWS?

As we saw in the last chapter, participant observation should always be the first choice for qualitative research, if it is possible and practicable. The data that you get from observation only goes through one layer of transformation before you start analysing it – as you select what to record and write it down or transcribe it. The same is broadly true of documents, as we will see in the next chapter. Interview data always goes through at least two layers of transformation, and often three. The first is when the interviewer chooses the question to ask. The second is when the informant creates an answer that shapes their experience to fit the question. The third is where the interviewer proposes possible answers, signalling what they expect, or the informant tries to infer what the interviewer wants to hear from them. If you are not clear about this, look back to our brief introduction to conversation analysis at the end of Chapter 6. Interviews have the same three-turn structure as every other form of interaction between two people.

Having said this, there are, of course, occasions when it is sensible and appropriate to use interviews:

- *When you are asking people about settings that are difficult to observe because of their intimate or private nature* – In practice, there are few settings where it is impossible to observe, and observation has not been done at some time. Confession in the Catholic Church and debates in the British Cabinet are the only ones that come immediately to mind. Participant observers have lived with families, loitered in public toilets watching gay sex, and stood beside pathologists as they dissected human bodies. Nevertheless, as a student, you do not have the time and resources – and probably not the access – to negotiate your way into such settings, let alone get ethics approval for your work.
- *When you are asking about events that have happened in the past* – This might be the immediate past, if you are asking people about what happened on a shift when you were not working or were not scheduled to observe. Alternatively, you might want to ask patients about how they came to be in a hospital bed or a clinic. What happened to bring them there? The past might be more remote, as social science interviews shade into oral history. Perhaps you want to ask retired nurses about their memories of work or training at the beginning of their careers.
- *When you want to ask your informants about their internal states of mind, motivations or emotions* – What were you thinking when this happened? Why did you choose to act in this way rather than that way? What were your feelings while you were carrying out those actions – and afterwards? These are particularly tricky questions and we shall say more about them later in this chapter.
- *When time and money are short* – As we have noted, participant observation can be slow and costly, although more rapid methods have been proposed and used. Provided you are careful with your analysis, interviews can give you useful data that are more likely than not to produce a sufficiently relevant answer to your questions for many practical purposes. Think of RD's example in Chapter 6 of the postdoc who was trying to get a more beautiful image of his bacteria for the purposes of publication. He did not need to do this. The Petri dish in front of him showed that his experiment worked but the expectations of his scientific peers led him to seek a more perfect demonstration. Do not make perfect science the enemy of useful science.

SELF-ASSESSMENT ACTIVITY

Should interviews be included in your research design?
  Ask yourself:

- Are there alternative ways of answering your research question through observation or documentary review?
- Do you have the time and other resources to carry out an observational study?
- Are the settings where you might find data relevant to your research question accessible to you?
- Are you clear about the possible biases and limitations of interviews?
- Are you aware of any ethical implications which may arise?

WHAT KIND OF INTERVIEW SHOULD YOU DO?

You can think of interviews as arranged along a continuum. At one end are the highly-structured interviews that are used in survey research and opinion polls. They may take place over the telephone or virtually over the Internet, as well as face to face. The interviewer, real or virtual, has a script that they are expected to follow. The wording of the questions, their sequence and the possible responses are determined in advance. At the other end we would find the natural interviews that we discussed in the previous chapter, opportunist questions intended to gather more information about how and why something happened during participant observation. In between we have an array of more or less structured interviews: they may be described as in-depth, non-directive, informal, open-ended, narrative, naturalistic, ethnographic or conversational. The most common labels are probably *semi-structured* or *unstructured*.

The last term is a bit misleading – remember our quote from Burgess. If an interview is a 'conversation with a purpose', then it must have some sort of a structure for that purpose to be achieved – which is why the label 'non-directive' is also confusing. Interviews simply vary in the degree to which that structure is made formal and visible. You might plan the interview in some detail, working out the sequence of topics and the question wording. In the actual interview, you might adjust the sequence or wording as the conversation flows or you learn the words the informant likes to use. Think of all the different ways in which nurses ask patients if they are passing urine regularly and easily, for example. Planning at this level of detail can help less experienced people feel more secure.

On the other hand, you can just go into an interview with a list of topics you want to cover and check them off as they come up. Informants may suggest new topics which you can add to the agenda for future interviews. This requires more skill, although you could probably carry it off if you are looking at a context you already know quite a lot about. If you have worked in transplant nursing, for example, and you want to find out more about how nurses manage the families of organ donors, you are likely to have a good idea of what it would be important to ask and how best to do that. The challenge would be making sure that you were also asking questions that could produce answers you did not expect to get. This is why qualitative interviews are sometimes described as 'in-depth', although this is another deceptive label – does anyone set out to do a 'superficial' or 'shallow' interview?

—————— VIDEO SUPPORT ——————

To see an example of how a researcher organised and explained their own research, view Keenan's (2018) video *Researching Nurse Educators: Lessons Learned From a Phenomenological Approach* in which she explains the aim of her research, her research methods, and lessons learned throughout the research. You can access the video by visiting this book's online resources: https://study.sagepub.com/dingwallandstaniland.

A variant form of qualitative interviewing is the group interview or *focus group* where participants are brought together to discuss a topic of interest to the researcher. You might, for example, assemble a group of patients with a chronic illness to talk about the ways in which they manage this in everyday life or about their encounters with health professionals. The participants may stimulate each other's stories and you can collect a lot of data quickly. These are reasons why this is quite a popular technique, especially among survey researchers who are looking for sound bites to illustrate their statistical reports. However, they do need careful management and analysis to ensure that all the participants get to have their say and that you are clear who the audience is for any contribution. It is important to bear in mind whether this is being produced for you or for other members of the group. What are the transformations involved in these data? There may also be ethical issues: how far should you encourage people to talk in front of an audience about highly personal issues, or about third parties who are not in the room? Should you protect people from their own disclosures or be concerned about the anonymity and privacy of people who are not there to speak for themselves?

Recently, there has also been some interest in using social media for qualitative research. You might create a page somewhere, possibly with a template like an interview agenda, and invite people to post their responses, drawing attention to your page by posts on platforms like Twitter, Instagram or TikTok. If you are interested in doing this, you should discuss it carefully with your supervisor. How much will you be able to trust that people are who they say they are? Will the posts be visible to everyone? If so, what about the expectations of privacy that we have already suggested might be problematic for focus groups? Remember, too, that the terms of service on many platforms mean that the company owns the data. This may have an impact on your ability to write about it and, possibly, publish it. It certainly has implications about any promises that you give informants about who can access the data and how confidentially it will be handled.

Ultimately, your decision about what kind of interviews to do and how far to structure them should be guided by your experience, your research questions and the current state of knowledge about the topics. If you are exploring a local problem in the context of a substantial body of existing knowledge from elsewhere, then you might use a more structured approach and concentrate on identifying local similarities and differences to the findings from elsewhere. How can you best locate your case relative to others so that you can draw on the general body of theory that has been created?

On the other hand, if very little has previously been written on the topic, you may need to adopt a more exploratory approach. Many hospitals, for example, have been introducing new roles for nurses in liaison between health and social care. If you were studying these, your questions might be quite general in order to find out exactly what their work consists of. Once you understand this, you might focus the questions rather more: there is, for example, a body of potentially relevant previous research by people who have studied other organisations looking at boundary-spanning roles.

Key Point

- Interviews and focus groups are the most common techniques of data collection used in qualitative health care research.
- Interviews can be used to explore the views, experiences, beliefs and motivations of individual participants.
- Focus groups use the interactions between their participants, in addition to the interactions between individuals and the researcher, to generate qualitative data.

DECIDING WHO TO TALK TO

Your thinking about what kind of interview to do might also be influenced by your decisions about who you want to talk to. What kind of *sample* do you want to create? Quantitative researchers usually want to create a sample that is *representative* of a defined population. This is how opinion polls work, where surveys of a few thousand people can give reasonably accurate estimates of the thinking of tens of millions of people. The sample is intended to represent the population in terms of key variables like age, gender, ethnicity, sexual orientation, marital status, level of education and so on. Quantitative researchers have various ways of creating representative samples, and adjusting the results for any significant gaps or shortfalls in the recruitment of people to match the key variables. Qualitative researchers rarely work on the same scale but may sometimes want to have a sample that is representative of the smaller groups that they are dealing with. If you are studying primary care nurses in a small city, for example, you might try to get a list of names and interview every fifth person on that list, in exactly the same way as a survey researcher might.

More commonly, qualitative researchers will either want to create a *theoretical* sample or to interview everyone connected with the case they are interested in.

A **theoretical sample** has much the same logic as that of critical experiments in fields like chemistry or engineering. You think about the features of a case that seem to be interesting or important and then deliberately set out to test them.

Definition

In RD's child protection study, for example, the main fieldwork site was a relatively affluent county with a small city surrounded by rural areas that attracted well-off residents. There were only a few pockets of poverty, especially around military bases. The attractions of the area meant there was little difficulty in recruiting professional staff in health, social care and legal services. When the team were offered funds to extend their work, they had a discussion about what would contrast with this site and present critical tests for their analysis. They selected a poor, remote and sparsely populated rural area and a rustbelt area whose heavy industry was rapidly disappearing. (With even more funds, they would have added an ethnically diverse inner-city area.) The logic was that, if the provisional conclusions reached from the main site were applicable to such contrasting cases, there was a plausible argument for claiming that they would be generally true of child protection work in England. Within each comparative area, the team then tried to interview people in roles that matched those they had shadowed in the main site.

You can follow the same process at an individual level. Suppose you want to find out how nurses keep up with research and whether this reflects their prior education. You might talk to some nurses who graduated from elite schools, contrast them with graduates from non-elite schools, and, in the future, with nurses from degree apprenticeships. You might also want to include some nurses who had received their main education outside the UK. This process of comparison and contrast is a way to develop more robust conclusions than just talking to people from any one group. For a shorter project, you might use published work as a point of contrast. Perhaps you read a paper about gender issues in nursing and realise that the author only talked to female nurses. You could take the same questions, or adapt them, and ask them of male nurses. Although you have only talked to men, you have the data on women for comparison. Remember what we said about putting bricks in the wall.

Key Point

The most important thing about deciding who to talk to is that it is a decision, and that you know why you have taken it: there will be a *purpose* in *this* conversation with *this* person.

PREPARING FOR AN INTERVIEW

For anything other than a natural interview, your preparations will need to deal with two sets of issues: logistic and scientific. How are you going to organise the interview, and how are you going to get useful and relevant information out of it? Although getting the right data is the most important objective, we are going to begin by saying a few things about setting up interviews because these practical concerns are often overlooked. However, if you do not get them right, you will find it hard to recruit informants and get the information you need.

—————————————— VIDEO SUPPORT ——————————————

It may be useful, at this stage, to watch *Research Participant Recruitment: Planning for a Recruitment Phase*, in order to consider the advantages of collecting data through qualitative measures and examine difficulties that can arise with recruitment. You can access the video by visiting this book's online resources: https://study.sagepub.com/dingwallandstaniland.

ORGANISING THE INTERVIEW

Your starting point has to be that the informant is doing you a favour. Nobody *has* to agree to an interview. As we were writing this chapter, we saw a tweet from someone who had been asked to take part in a clinical trial of a new treatment for haemophilia. This would have involved weekly attendance at a clinic for monitoring, taking about five hours end to end. As the tweeter asked, who could fit this into a normal working life? Was he supposed to use up his annual leave? The researchers had only thought about what was convenient for them. As a result, he had refused to participate. There is an important lesson here for all researchers: make it easy for people to take part in your project. For the duration of the data collection at least, your convenience definitely takes second place. If you have domestic or caring responsibilities, you need to think about how you will manage any potential conflicts.

    The standard advice is to choose a place where you can be undisturbed and talk to the informant in a relatively private way. It should be somewhere that is easy for them to access and where they will feel relaxed. This is good advice – but you should also recognise when it doesn't work. If you interview someone in a room in a hospital or on a university campus, your informant may feel less comfortable than you do. Many people find these very strange and unsettling places. Doing an interview in someone's home may be more comfortable for them, but it may also be hard to talk privately. Sometimes, the best answer may be to talk in a café, a pub or a community centre. Where people are comfortable with technology, you could think of doing an interview by telephone or over the Internet using a video calling service. Your university will probably have a standard choice of software for this. You also need to be realistic with informants about how much of their time you will need.

While your informant's convenience comes first, you should also give some attention to your own safety. Are you putting yourself at risk by going to other people's houses or to meeting places in an unfamiliar neighbourhood? In Chapter 5 we referred to the PhD managed by RD where a woman student was interviewing men with a record of violence towards their partners and how she developed a protection plan. Most social research comes with some risk, and we have sometimes seen a rather macho indifference to this by both students and supervisors. We cannot eliminate risks completely without cutting ourselves off from important knowledge. This does not, though, mean we should not try to manage them.

However you decide to handle these practical matters, you should keep a detailed note of your decisions and include this in the report of your research. When your readers are assessing your findings, it is important that they know the context in which they were produced. How might this have shaped the talk between you and your informant? What influence did it have on the way your informant saw you and what they thought they should say in response to your questions?

PLANNING THE INTERVIEW

We have stressed the importance of being clear what you want to achieve from an interview. This is the point at which you should look back at your research question and your literature review and write down a list of objectives. When you have completed the interview, what information do you want to have collected? This does not mean you should ignore other things that come up. Most interview agendas evolve as they are used. You will discover that some of your topics are meaningless or irrelevant to your informants – and that they want to talk about some things that you had not thought about. If this happens, you will need to revise the plan, so you ask a reasonably consistent set of questions from all or most of your informants. You may want to retain some of your own topics so you can explore why they do not make sense to your informants, but you should certainly be ready to add in new ones which seem more important to them.

This plan should then be compressed into an agenda for the interview. Ideally, this should be no more than one side of A4 or one screen on a tablet or laptop computer. This is so you can see the whole of the interview at a single glance and keep track of topics if they come up out of order. We still like to use paper for agendas because it is easy to tick off topics or scribble ideas as they come up – perhaps noting a point to come back to later in the interview. We print a new sheet for each interview and file it with our notes or transcripts as a record of what we did at the time. However, there is software that will do a similar job and you may prefer to use that. The compression of the plan should reduce it to a set of prompts for yourself – they may just be key words or phrases to remind you of the objective. You may also want to suggest some model questions to yourself, especially if you do not feel very confident. With practice, you will probably find you ignore these, but they are useful to have in reserve.

HOW DO YOU ASK USEFUL QUESTIONS?

Interviews generally involve a mixture of several types of questions, which may be used at different stages for different purposes.

These are some of the main types of question:

- Demographic or scene-setting questions are often used at the beginning of an interview. They are quite factual and 'obvious' so they help to relax the informant and encourage them to feel confident in talking to the interviewer:
  - o 'Perhaps we might begin by you taking me through your career and how you came to be doing this job?'
  - o 'I know we are here mainly to talk about this baby, but can I just ask whether you have any other children and how old you were when you had them?'
- Closed questions are intended to elicit a yes/no/don't know response when you want to know something quite specific. Although they are more common in survey interviews, they still have a place in qualitative interviews:
  - o 'Do you have a copy of the policy/guideline/protocol for treating patients with this condition?'
  - o 'Did you go to the briefing meeting last week about the new triage system in A&E?'
- Direct questions are related to closed questions. They are most useful when you are asking your informant to teach you about something:
  - o 'How is this treatment supposed to manage leg ulcers?'
  - o 'What does this test result tell you about the patient's condition?'
- Open questions are used to ask more generally about behaviours, feelings or experiences:
  - o 'What do you think are the benefits of the involvement of staff with this policy?'
  - o 'From your own experience, what do you think of that?'
  - o 'How did that make you feel?'
- Although open questions are very common in qualitative interviews, they can be difficult to analyse because they are so general. This makes them particularly vulnerable to the desire of your informants to say the 'right thing', whatever they think that may be. You may, of course, want to find out what people think they are supposed to say, which can be interesting and relevant data. However, you probably want to try to anchor these general questions more closely in specific events. If we take the three examples above, we might sometimes want to accompany them with *specifying* questions like these:
  - o 'Can you give me an example of when there was a benefit from staff involvement with the policy?'
  - o 'When was the last time you had that experience …?'
  - o 'Have there been any occasions when that happened, and you did not feel like that?'
- Prompt questions are similar to specifying questions but may be used at any point to encourage informants to give more information or elaborate their answers:
  - o 'That's interesting; please can you tell me more about that?'

   o   'How do you think that relates to …?'
   o   'Why do you think that is?'

Across the course of an interview, questions usually 'funnel' the informant from broad generalities to more specific and detailed concerns. This may happen across the whole of the interview or within each of the main topics that you have identified. There are some techniques that can help you with this.

VIDEO SUPPORT

There are many videos available giving qualitative interviewing tips. One such is *Interview Guide (Qualitative Interviews #2)*. You can access the video by visiting this book's online resources: https://study.sagepub.com/dingwallandstaniland.

GROUNDING TECHNIQUES

The attempt to manage the problem of the relationship between what people say and what they do – or in the case of an interview, how they describe what they have done – has led to various innovations in qualitative interviews. Three of these are worth mentioning here:

1   *Vignettes* are short scenarios, in written, pictorial or video form, that try to describe actual examples of events and what people did about them. They are 'stories about individuals, situations and structures which can make reference to important points in the study of perceptions, beliefs and attitudes' (Hughes, 1998: 381). They are quite useful as an alternative to specifying questions because they may be less threatening. Informants are asked to talk about fictional events rather than real ones. If you look back to the example in Chapter 6 of KS's silence about the doctor who did not wash his hands, you should be able to see that this is linked to the scenario of the phlebotomist who dropped a cannula in Chapter 5. KS was willing to disclose her choice, which might not be one other nurses would have made, but the vignette offers an alternative way to explore such decisions.

Key Point

Vignettes are useful for three main purposes in social research:

- To allow actions in context to be explored.
- For clarification of judgements.
- To provide a less personal and therefore less threatening way of exploring sensitive topics.

2   *Talking with records* involves having the informant sit with a case file and go through it with the interviewer. The informant can be asked to expand on the record entries and to explain how particular decisions came to be made at specific points in the case. RD used this technique quite extensively in his child protection research to validate the conclusions from two years' observational work in the main study site through three-week visits to the comparator sites. Although a small amount of observation was done in each site, the core data came from social workers and health visitors talking him through selected case files. This anchored the data closely in their actual practice and the workings of their organisations and the interagency system that is involved in dealing with child abuse and neglect.

3   *Digital storytelling* is attracting increasing interest. In the most elaborate versions, informants collaborate in making three-to five-minute videos about their lives, using photos, participant voices, drawings and music. Simpler versions might just create posters, portfolios, scrapbooks or albums that present the informant's images of key events and experiences. The researcher is a 'facilitator' in these creative processes (Lenette et al., 2015). These storytelling techniques can increase the engagement of participants with a research project and present a different perspective on its core questions. They can also be used as an alternative to 'talking with records' as prompts for answers grounded in experience. Advocates claim that these techniques are particularly useful in gaining an understanding of the more emotional dimensions of health work and health care. This technique does require a degree of skill in using digital media production equipment and software. If suitable training, editing facilities and hardware are not available, you may be better using lower-technology tools to make static representations in posters and so on.

LISTENING IS IMPORTANT

So far, we have focused on how to get your informant to talk and to tell you about the things you are interested in. Before we move on, though, we should remind you about the importance of listening. There are two aspects to this.

First, one of the commonest mistakes made by less experienced researchers is asking the next question too quickly. You have to learn how not to be worried by silence. If your informant stops talking, do not ask the next question immediately. Pause for a few beats to see whether they have more to say. Very often, your informant is trying to judge your response and to decide whether they have said enough or whether you would like to hear something more. Sometimes, they are working out whether to trust you with more sensitive information than they gave you at the start. You do not have to hold back to the extent that your silence becomes oppressive or embarrassing – but you do not need to rush in with the next question.

Second, keep showing your informant that you are listening to their answers to your questions. This is one of the features that makes an interview a little different from ordinary conversation. Refer back explicitly to previous answers: 'A few moments ago, you said that…, could we come back to that topic …?' Use your informant's first name from time to time, if this is appropriate. Pick up the informant's choice of words or phrases. Is there some hospital slang or technical vocabulary you can probe?

> 'You said that the response to that cardiac arrest was a bit of a "Code Hollywood"? Do you often get these, where it feels like putting on a show rather than seriously expecting a result?'

Your body language and eye contact are also important in showing how fascinated you are by what the informant has to say but your understanding of how conversations work is probably your most powerful tool.

At the beginning, we noted how interview skills could feed back into your clinical practice: the art of listening is one skill that many health professionals do not develop to a high enough level. Research interviews are great opportunities to improve your listening and reflection on what your patients are actually saying to you.

Key Point

An interview agenda can act as a prompt, reminding you of necessary topics to cover, questions to ask and areas to probe. It should be simple so that your primary focus can stay on the respondent. Ideally it is best to memorise any agenda, but if you are an inexperienced interviewer it may help to:

- *Write down* the larger research questions of the study and then outline the ranges of knowledge relevant to answering these questions.
- *Develop questions* within each major area, shaping them to fit with respondents' expertise and experience.
- *Think about* a logical flow to the interview.
- *Begin the interview with* some 'warm-up' questions to build rapport with the informant.
- *Ask 'how' questions rather than 'why' questions* to capture processes rather than descriptions of behaviour: 'How did you come to be a nurse …?'
- *Elicit more detailed and elaborate responses* by building on the informant's answers to your key questions.

Try to provide closure with a last question to leave the respondent feeling empowered and listened to.

RECORDING THE ANSWERS

Many of the things we said in the last chapter about recording observations also apply to interviews. Although most people use an audio recorder these days, you should always think about whether this is justifiable. Audio recordings do give you a great deal more detail and allow you to defend the accuracy of your quotes. However, you must allow for the time you will spend transcribing them when planning the project. This will depend upon the level of detail you need. Transcription is an important constraint on sample size in qualitative research – it is costly in somebody's time. As a student that is probably yours! A basic, usable transcript requires about 3–4 hours of work for each hour of recording. If you are interested in a more detailed analysis of the interaction between yourself and the informant, transcription may take two or three times as long. In practice, researchers often listen to a replay, make notes and then select which passages need to be transcribed in greater detail.

You should also remember that some informants may feel threatened by the use of a recorder, particularly if they are discussing stigmatised or unlawful behaviour or experiences. In some situations, recording may be difficult just because of the surrounding sound levels. If you are meeting an informant in a café, for example, you may not be able to distinguish your interactions from all the other talk that is going on.

Taking notes during an interview is always good practice, whatever you decide about recording. If the technology fails because you have forgotten to charge the recorder or put in fresh batteries, you may still be able to recapture key passages from the interview. Your informant may also see your note-taking as evidence of your interest in what they have to say. You are not just doing the interview on auto-pilot but are really engaged with it. Your notes are also an opportunity to capture things that are not on the recording. Think ahead here. What will you need to know when you begin analysing the data? How will you evaluate what your informant has said to you? We shall say more about this when we come to discuss analysis in a later chapter. However, remember what we have said about the importance of reflecting on the interaction between researchers and the people they are researching. How you are perceived shapes the answers that your informants give you. They are making an assessment of what responses will make them appear to you to be reasonable, rational, ethical and in all respects competent to be doing what they are doing. As we noted in the previous chapter, they are *giving accounts* rather than *literal descriptions* of what they might be thinking or feeling, or what their motives were, in doing whatever they have done (Dingwall, 1997). However sensitive and gentle our interview techniques may be, they cannot be expected to neutralise informants' awareness of the ways in which their behaviour could be judged and found wanting. Their responses will be constrained by the need to rebut any negative evaluation that their actions might attract. Interviews only collect the accounts that are produced for the interviewer. You can try to control this to some degree by the techniques of grounding that we described, but you cannot eliminate this dimension of your data.

Treating your informants' talk as accounts will allow you to explore how informants define their motivations, knowledge and experiences in ways that they think are relevant to the research questions being asked. It is, nevertheless, still possible in skilful qualitative research interviewing to challenge an informant's perspective.

—————————————— FREEING OUR IMAGINATION ——————————————

Challenging an informant

Watch the following exchange of *US President Trump's Clash with CNN's Jim Acosta* from November 2018 – you can access the video by visiting this book's online resources: https://study.sagepub.com/dingwallandstaniland. Consider what you could do if this happened to you.

Research users should expect to see interview data interpreted in relation to the context in which it was produced. Analyses should start from the question of what informants can be seen to be doing with their interview talk. They must consider the complexity, instability and ambivalence that is characteristic of informants' understandings. This approach points the way to another use to which interview data may be put: as a source of data on the expected behaviour in the context that your informants are telling you about.

If you are to allow for this properly in your analysis, you need to make your data as transparent as you can. Your transcripts or notes should reconstruct people's actual words – including your questions – rather than summarising or editing them. You may do that later when you are writing up, but you must be able to show a chain of evidence back to the original interaction if you ever need to. You should also have a note about the context of the interview – where and when did it take place? Were there any disruptions? How engaged did the informant seem to be? What do you think they made of you? In the same way as many participant observers keep a parallel record of their reflections on each session of fieldwork, you may find it useful to have two records of each interview: one trying to capture the event itself as accurately as you can, and the other trying to preserve your own experience of it and any thoughts that may be useful in later analysis.

Qualitative interviews have made a significant contribution to health studies. Sometimes, such interviews may be the method of choice. They provide data on locations and social processes which would not otherwise be open to investigation. This may be because the phenomenon of interest to a researcher does not occur in a focused and identifiable location that would permit observation or because it occurs in a situation that is private or one to which access is blocked. Interviews offer opportunities to investigate different professional participants' understandings, especially if, for example, there is a breakdown in communication, which results from a lack of appreciation of other perspectives. Qualitative interviews can be a way of uncovering different perspectives and of exposing each group to the thinking of the others.

Qualitative research interviews can also offer an escape route from some of the more obstinate problems and inconsistencies that beset quantitative forms of interviewing. The data they elicit can undermine the taken-for-granted assumptions of researchers and policy-makers. In doing so, they offer the opportunity to discover aspects of a policy-relevant issue or problem which could not have been predicted at the outset of a study.

Nevertheless, the potential of qualitative interviews will not be fully exploited unless researchers take a sophisticated approach to the analysis of data. When interviews are used to generate reports on external realities, this must rest on conscientious and explicitly reflexive assessments of the data. Where they are used to elicit accounts of informants' internal realities, analysis must be sensitive to the interactional and political contexts in which the data were generated. In this way researchers will guard against drawing superficial conclusions about the motives and meanings of health care providers and recipients.

These problems of analysis are not unique to interviews and we shall return to them when we have looked at our third qualitative method, reading the papers.

CHAPTER SUMMARY POINTS

This chapter has addressed the many aspects of interviewing in qualitative research.

Qualitative interviews explore how informants describe their experiences and practices as these are relevant to the core research questions. However, these descriptions are both a reflection of the external reality of the world and of the informant's state of mind. The challenge that you will come to later is to work out which is which during any particular passage of the interview. The skilful use of qualitative interviews is one way to bring out the ways in which informants use the beliefs and understandings that we might call their *culture* to recapture and make sense of events and experiences.

Treating interviews as social interactions, where everyone – interviewer and informant alike – is trying to produce contextually-appropriate behaviours has fundamental implications. Interviews do not simply report on mental states that underlie behaviour. They are occasions where informants – and interviewers – offer accounts for their actions, feelings and opinions. In providing these accounts both parties would normally seek to present themselves as knowledgeable and, indeed, decent members of a community – as acceptable parents, good patients, well-informed citizens, accountable adults and competent professionals – or to offer a socially acceptable explanation of failure.

FURTHER READING

This chapter has cited several helpful sources for further reading about interview methods. If you want to know more specifically about focus groups, this is a good place to start:

Bloor, M.J, Frankland, J., Thomas, M. and Robson, K. (2000) *Focus Groups in Social Research*. London: Sage.

Helen Kara, an experienced freelance qualitative researcher, has produced a nice introduction to the idea of a 'conversation with a purpose' in graphic art format:

Kara, H. and Jackson, S. (2018) *Conversation with a Purpose*. Available at https://drhelenkara.files.wordpress.com/2018/06/conversation-with-a-purpose.pdf (accessed 28/2/20).

These are two useful discussions of the use of qualitative interviews in health care settings:

Dicicco-Bloom, B. and Crabtree, B.F. (2006) 'The qualitative research interview', *Medical Education*, 40(4): 314–21. Available at https://onlinelibrary.wiley.com/doi/full/10.1111/j.1365-2929.2006.02418.x (accessed 28/2/20).

Hunt, M.R., Chan, L.S. and Mehta, A. (2011) 'Transitioning from clinical to qualitative research interviewing', *International Journal of Qualitative Methods*, September: 191–201. Available at https://doi.org/10.1177/160940691101000301 (accessed 28/2/20).

8

Analysing Documents and Artefacts

Learning Outcomes

At the end of this chapter you will be able to:

- Demonstrate the historical importance of analysing documents and artefacts
- Discuss the interaction between work and documents
- Recognise how artefacts create internal and external representations of organisations
- Discuss key strategies for data exploration using different types of documents
- Introduce the social construction of organisational statistics
- Give an example of a social construction of document analysis

Humans have been creating representations of themselves and their everyday activities for at least forty thousand years. All around the world, caves were painted with hunting scenes, images of animals, and handprints from the artists and other members of the group to which they belonged. Social scientists who specialise in the study of early humans puzzle over precisely what the artists were trying to achieve. What do these artefacts tell us about the people who produced them and how they wanted to be seen, by themselves and others?

With the development of literacy and numeracy around ten thousand years ago, the possibilities for creating representations were dramatically expanded. Social groups were able to keep records of their activities and to define their meaning in ways that had not previously been possible. When a society depends mainly on oral communication, its history is what people can remember.

Such societies develop ways of making themselves easily memorable – but memories are fallible, fluid and open to adjustment. Writing and other forms of recording mean that you can check memories: think of US President Donald Trump denying that he described the Duchess of Sussex as 'nasty', when you can listen to the audio recording of him doing just that. Health care records document patients' lives and join up their contacts with all the different professionals who write in them. Qualitative research is interested in the patients' stories and in *what* we can learn from *who* gets to contribute to them in *what* ways. How do documents, which may be paper or computer files, relate to the work of health care providers?

Another category of documents is produced by nations, institutions and organisations to create an image of themselves that they would like to be known by. Remember in the previous chapter when we discussed how interviews were occasions when informants tried to represent themselves as reasonable, rational and moral people? The same is true of social groups. If a hospital is trying to recruit staff, it will produce documents that portray it as a good employer, regardless of the actual experience of its current workers. Looking at these documents helps us to understand how the hospital management would like to be seen by key audiences. Although we are talking about 'documents' here, we could actually think of a wide range of artefacts.

Definition

By an **artefact**, we mean something, material or virtual, that is the product of human creativity.

Older hospitals, for example, often have statues, honours boards, stained glass windows and the like, which were intended to impress their sponsors with the seriousness of purpose to be found in the institution. Modern hospitals have hi-tech atriums, borrowing designs from airports and luxury hotels to signal their commitment to cutting-edge, personalised care. Think of the elaborate coding of traditional nursing uniforms, with echoes of religious orders and visible markers of experience and seniority in stripes and badges. How does this compare with wearing scrubs that make few distinctions between different professions and grades of worker?

Some of these documents will now be virtual, like hospital websites. How do these represent the hospital to potential patients? Are there differences between public and private hospitals? Are the websites accessible to people with a range of sensory disabilities? What does it say about an organisation if they are not?

Other documents measure the activities of societies, and of the organisations that we find within them. One of the first uses of numeracy was to create accounts for royal households, merchant traders and state granaries. In our own time, the description of nations, institutions and organisations in numerical terms has become a major industry. That industry, however, often takes the numbers for granted. Qualitative researchers look at how the numbers are created in the first place, and then at how they become the basis for the development of policies and professional practices. Is 50 per cent of a glass of water half-full or half-empty? The number itself does not tell you.

Of course, your own research is also producing a lot of documents in the form of the reflective notes, field notes, recordings and summaries that you have been collecting as we went through the book. Understanding how documents work will contribute to creating your own, as we shall discuss in the next chapter. However, it is also a core professional skill. Wherever you go in practice, you will need to compile records of your actions, understand the quantitative reports that are produced by your employer, read published research, or write reports intended to persuade other people to adopt your preferred view of a person, event or situation.

This chapter then, will look at three broad topics in relation to documents and other artefacts: the interaction between work and documents; the internal and external representation of organisations; and the social construction of organisational statistics. We will work through some case studies and then finish by drawing out some general principles that you could use when looking at documents.

WHY STUDY DOCUMENTS?

Document analysis is often under-valued as a form of qualitative research, particularly for undergraduates, but it provides a rich source of data. Documents have real consequences. Ask yourself: Who writes them? Who reads them? How should they be read? How are they used? A focus on documents is particularly valuable if time and resources are limited:

- It can be efficient and effective. Locating and analysing documents is often far more cost efficient and time efficient than conducting your own research or experiments (Bowen, 2009). Also, documents are stable, 'non-reactive' data sources, meaning that they can be read and reviewed multiple times and remain unchanged by the researcher's influence or research process (2009: 31).
- Except for personal medical or employment records, document studies are unlikely to raise issues for ethics committees. Many documents are already in the public domain or deal with information that may be sensitive for an organisation but not for individual patients or employees. Once terms of access have been agreed, documents can quickly be used in a study.
- Where documents are not already public, they are relatively easy to anonymise. While each hospital has some unique organisational features, the requirements of external funders or regulators mean that they need to produce broadly similar statistics, records and reports to describe and justify their activities and expenditure. The same would be true for primary care centres, public health services and private clinics.
- Where documents are public, they are also easy to share. Readers can have their own independent access to your sources in order to check your analysis and findings. In this respect, they are different from most field notes or interviews, where your first duty is to protect the anonymity and confidentiality of your informants rather than sharing the data with all comers.

- Document analysis can supplement other qualitative methods. Documents can provide contextual or background information for observations. They may also contain data that no longer can be observed, provide details that informants have forgotten, and track changes and developments. These may prompt questions for interviews and help to encourage your informants to connect their answers to specific events rather just giving you general statements (Bowen, 2009).

SOME GENERAL ISSUES

The first thing to remember about any document, or other artefact, is that it was produced in a social context by one person, or group of people, in order to make a particular impression on another person or group of people and generate some further action or response from them. In the course of this process, documents can become detached from the actions that created them and come to be seen as more objective and factual than, for example, the accounts given by their authors in interviews, which are 'mere personal belief' (Hammersley and Atkinson, 2019:133). Once something is put on paper, or into a database, its history can be forgotten.

CASE STUDY SCENARIO

Sally Macintyre (1978) was studying the management of pregnancy in a large maternity hospital. When women came for their first consultation, the midwives filled in a very long form, with questions that often frustrated both the midwives and the women using the service. Macintyre observed how the midwives and the women worked together to invent answers to the questions that would allow them to get through the process quickly and smoothly. Some months later, however, she also observed a feedback session where the midwives were presented with the statistics that had been generated from these forms. The audience were impressed by what the numbers revealed about their work and the women they had booked into the hospital. As Macintyre noted, the improvisation that had gone into the completion of the forms had been forgotten and the statistics were treated as an objective description of the clinic and its users. Although this is quite an old study, our own experiences suggest that very little has changed. RD was recently (2019) a patient in an A&E department. One of the first questions that he was asked was his date of birth, which is the way the health service distinguishes between people who might share the same names. However, before being discharged, the doctor who had been treating him realised that he had not completed the online form correctly. He returned to ask about RD's smoking and drinking habits – where clearly any answer could have been given – and whether RD knew when it was his birthday and what day of the week it was. This last was obviously intended as some kind of mental status assessment, which was rather redundant, given that it had been preceded by detailed clinical discussions about the medical emergency and its management. Nevertheless, the form had to be filled in – and 'Yes, I do know when my birthday is' was not a sufficient answer! Indeed, you might wonder who had the memory problem here, given that the very same information had already been provided in a slightly different form about an hour earlier. Nevertheless, the discharge could not occur until the 'correct' answers had been provided. You might also notice that the question assumed that RD came from a cultural background where birthdays and memorable dates were important.

We shall look at some more examples of these processes later. For the moment, however, the important thing to remember is that, although documents may appear to be 'facts', they are always part of a story of *creation* and *interpretation*. Documentary analysis tells that story and helps us understand how the documents come to be treated as factual and what this might mean for their understanding and use (ten Have, 2004). Do they incorporate particular, selective ways of assembling the information that they convey as they present a '*documentary reality*' (Atkinson and Coffey, 1997:47, our italics)?

Garfinkel (1967: 197–207) showed that clinical records were *contractual* rather than *actuarial*. This means that they did not describe what had happened in a *literal* way but provided *accounts* – evidence that the people who wrote them had done their work in a competent and professional manner. How does this shape our understanding of the world, particularly when quantitative research, organisational management and clinical practice often take the objectivity of records for granted?

DOCUMENTS AND WORK

CRITICAL THINKING EXERCISE

Make a list of all the documents you use in your day-to-day activities in health care (hard or electronic). Then make another list of all the document reference material that you *could/should* refer to for advice to support your everyday activity. Do they match? If not, why do you think this is?

One of the most important recent bodies of qualitative research on nursing has been produced by Davina Allen and her various collaborators. She has had a long-standing interest in the relationship between documents and everyday work. Some of her early publications (Allen, 1998, 2002), from her own PhD thesis, looked at the way in which nursing records had changed with the introduction of an approach to nursing termed the 'nursing process' from the US (Dingwall et al., 1988). This was a nurse-led change that also had implications for the way in which nurses recorded their work. It involved the creation of individual care plans based on four phases: assessment, planning, implementation and evaluation. Allen showed how these documents, originally intended to support individualised patient care and professional judgements by nurses, had become tools for quality assurance, led by hospital managers. Where they had previously been *actuarial* documents, intended for nurses to check their own practice, they had now become *contractual* documents, intended to show that the hospital had delivered care in a manner acceptable to external reviewers. Nurses described, for example, how they had been instructed to record 'bowels' and 'health education' as problems, regardless of whether they were or were not appropriate for the patient. Some wards had standardised texts for care plans that were simply copied for all patients. The result was that the nurses developed alternative, and less formal, documents for managing their work, particularly ward diaries and handover notes. The documents created by the nursing process described a 'Potemkin Village' of individualised professional care that was unrelated to the practical work of the ward. You will no doubt come across some version of this transformation in your own work!

Allen (2014a) returned to these issues about fifteen years later in another study, in a different hospital, intended to better understand what nurses did all day. There is a great deal of talk about how modern nurses are no longer at the bedside, providing tender loving care to their patients. This image of nursing has been false for a long time. It goes back to the days when medical interventions were limited, patient stays could be quite lengthy and nursing care was critical to recovery. Before antibiotics, for example, there was, indeed, little that could be done for pneumonia other than mopping down the patient to reduce their body temperature and give them a better chance of fighting off the infection on their own. Nevertheless, the nurse at the bedside is a more powerful image than the nurse as a skilled technician, supporting active and intensive treatments. It is also contrasted with the nurse as the person in an office, carrying out administrative tasks. There are constant calls to reduce these and put the nurse back on the wards – like putting police officers back on the streets, even though this is an inefficient and ineffective way of fighting modern crimes.

Allen found that so-called administration was at the core of nursing work – and probably always had been. Nurses were the backbone of the hospital as an organisation as the people who had the greatest degree of continuity on any ward. They co-ordinated everyone else and managed the patient's journey from admission to discharge (see also Allen 2014b). Their work involved constant interactions with members of other professional and non-professional groups within and outside the hospital, informed by their knowledge of the patients on their ward. In the face of constant pressures to free up beds, their negotiations were critical to maintaining the flow of patients through the organisation.

Record systems had moved on and were now mostly electronic. However, they were no better designed to support the actual work of the nurses. Like most electronic record systems, they had been shaped to collect information for the benefit of the managers who had briefed the design-ers rather than to support the actual workflow at the front-line (Harper et al., 1997; Sellen and Harper, 2003). People were supposed to work to fit the system rather than the system being fitted to the people. As a result, the nurses used a variety of improvised or informal paper documents to co-ordinate their everyday work: small notebooks, scraps of paper stuffed into uniform pockets, or brief notes on handover sheets. They would puzzle over the similarly scrappy messages left by other professionals. The electronic records constantly lagged behind and were updated periodically as required to create a professional appearance. Allen makes similar comments on the Patient Status at a Glance White Boards (PSAGWB). These never tell you what is happening right now so that any professional coming on to the ward confirms the information directly with the nurses rather than relying on the board. As Allen points out, a tool intended to reduce such interruptions actu-ally increases nursing workloads because a neat PSAGWB was treated as an indicator of a well-run ward and time had to be devoted to making it look good. You might recall the 'old-school' ward sister that we met in Chapter 1 and her ideas about a tidy ward. Have things really changed that much? Is this telling us something more fundamental about hospitals and the pressures to 'look good' at all levels?

CRITICAL THINKING EXERCISE

Go back to the list of documents that you put together.

- Which ones are contractual and which ones are actuarial?
- Which ones do you *actually use* in the course of the day?
- Who reads these documents?
- Who writes them?
- Do you use any unofficial documents like a personal notebook?
- When do you use electronic records and when do you use paper records?

It is important to stress that describing records as 'contractual' rather than 'actuarial' does not mean that they are irrelevant or pointless. The challenge is to find out what the contract is and what the benefits might be. KS's own PhD (Staniland, 2008) is a good example of this. Her approach to the study of clinical governance in a large UK general hospital was strongly influenced by Carolyn Wiener's (2000) work on the rise of quality assurance in the US through its impact on two large general hospitals. Wiener had shown how the changing social and political environment of US health care had created increasing pressures for accountability in the way that it was delivered. Hospitals had developed elaborate and expensive internal systems of performance measurement so that they could be seen to be doing a good job and, hence, be eligible to receive various types of public or private insurance payments. The hospitals were periodically reviewed by accrediting teams, who examined the performance data and interviewed institutional representatives. Wiener described the work that went into preparation for such visits: drives to complete and update all records, coaching doctors and nurses so they would give the 'right' answers when they were interviewed, rewriting procedural manuals in the accrediting body's preferred format and so on. This was vital work because any failures would have a very severe impact on the hospital's income and its ability to stay in business.

The UK National Health Service was under similar pressures to show that it was giving safe and effective care that represented value for money, and had imported, adapted or copied many of the processes that Wiener described. KS found that her hospital had created an elaborate system of committees and working groups that generated a vast number of documents – which virtually nobody ever read. There were something like 150 policy documents setting out local practice guidelines, 21 additional documents on infection control and 76 patient group directives. However, the search function on the hospital intranet site did not identify them; in fact, the 'clinical governance' area of the site was not tagged under 'clinical governance' and did not appear in search results. Moreover, when she talked to ward staff, it emerged that the ward computers were not able to access these materials. The only time they were used seemed to be after adverse events when ward nurses needed to write a report that showed how they had acted in accordance with the policy all along. The hospital did little to inform staff about new or revised policies unless they happened to come up by chance at a training event. Membership of the various committees and working groups remained obscure, so there were few opportunities for ward-level input through their supposed representatives.

Now you might think that clinical governance in this hospital was an expensive way of not achieving very much. A lot of senior, and well-paid, people spent time attending meetings. There were the costs of a secretariat to draft and manage the documents. At the end of the process, however, this work was invisible to the people who were caring for patients on a day-to-day basis. Quality assurance had no apparent impact on the quality of care at that level. This was certainly KS's initial reaction. However, when she thought more deeply about what she had seen, and read more widely about how organisations work, she realised that she had been missing the point. This process was actually very successful – just not in the way that you might expect! The quality of the quality assurance documents led to regional and national awards that promoted the hospital. As the NHS moved towards more of a market in patients, this attracted referrals, so the hospital gained more income at the expense of competitors. It brought some additional direct investments and reduced its contributions to the central fund from which the NHS paid for litigation and compensation to patients injured by clinical negligence. You could say that clinical practice benefited from these extra resources, although this was quite an indirect process. The other party to these contractual documents was not the patient hoping for quality care but the external organisations who supplied reputation and funds to the hospital.

Of course, quality assurance cannot be completely separated from service quality. The most obvious example is the crisis at Mid Staffordshire Hospital (Francis, 2013). Like the hospital studied by KS, this had a very successful quality assurance system that led it to be one of the first hospitals to gain recognition as a Foundation Trust. This brought extra funding and operational freedom, but the quality of care was very poor. Although patients and their relatives recognised this, it took many years for their complaints to penetrate the assumption that good documents proved good service quality. The complaints were seen as one-off issues rather than as evidence of systemic failures.

What we want you to take away from this section is a concern to ask what documents are *doing* in an organisation, rather than taking them for granted. You might even find it helpful to think of the documents as being like another human party in any situation, actively shaping work and interactions between staff or between staff and patients rather than just passive pieces of paper or data entry screens.

CRITICAL THINKING EXERCISE

You have just read about how good documents can benefit a hospital, even if they do not have the intended outcomes. Can you think of any similar examples from your own experience? You might want to look back at Davina Allen's comments on the PSAGWB or RD's experience with the form-filling in A&E. Have you seen anything like that where you have worked – being expected to do things that looked good rather than contributing to your immediate work? Who are they supposed to 'look good' to?

What benefits might flow from that?

REPRESENTING AN ORGANISATION

In the previous section, we introduced the idea that documents might be important in understanding how a hospital, or other health care organisation, persuaded the people that it dealt with to think of it as a good partner, to trust it and to direct money or other resources towards it. In this section, we will look at some of the things that a hospital, or a profession, might do that are more deliberately intended to get people to think well of it. We are also going to widen our focus here from paper or electronic documents to think more broadly about other kinds of artefacts – buildings, statues, awards and so on. Our case study draws on the history of nursing, although its techniques are just as applicable to the ways in which nursing is represented today. Indeed, one of the things we want to bring out is the way in which people construct stories about the history of the profession, or about the organisations and health systems within which its members work, that makes their present state seem like an inevitable outcome of the past. Historians, of course, see the past as much more a matter of chance and contingency, where people have different choices available to them at any time and could have followed very different paths.

——————————— **FREEING OUR IMAGINATION** ———————————

Look around your hospital or college. Does it have statues, stained glass, buildings or wards named after famous people – if so, which ones? Are there awards that carry the names of people or organisations? Did your induction include some historical information about your college or hospital?

How do you feel about these? Do they have a place in today's modern health service?

When Florence Nightingale returned from the Crimea, she was hailed as a national heroine. Dozens of commemorative items were produced – figurines, medallions, prints, lamps and so on. They turn up regularly at antique dealers and auctions – a vintage Staffordshire pottery figure would cost you several hundred pounds. Public donations created a charity to support her work, which continues today. Her name was attached to schools of nursing, to scholarships, to prizes, to buildings and hospital wards. In 1915, a statue was erected in her honour in Waterloo Place, where it crosses Pall Mall, surrounded by some of the UK's most elite institutions. If you go to the shop at the Florence Nightingale museum in London, you can find the same sort of objects on sale today. These are all examples of artefacts. When something like this happens to a person, the real individual often gets lost behind the images. They have become a symbol or an *icon*. We can ask what they have been made to symbolise. What selections have been made from the historical record of that person's life and work? Why have some things been chosen and not others? What message is being communicated here?

——————————— **FREEING OUR IMAGINATION** ———————————

Can you identify some online images/information of Florence Nightingale memorabilia?

What forms do these images appear in? How many different formats can you find?

Can you write a caption commenting on their iconic aspects?

In 1964, Elvi Whittaker and Virginia Olesen (1964), social scientists working in the School of Nursing at the University of California, San Francisco, published a paper looking at the way in which the historical figure of Florence Nightingale had been turned into an icon by the nursing profession. They were influenced by anthropological work on the way in which members of clan groups in traditional societies signalled their common membership through shared stories about their descent from a common ancestor. The ancestor figure stayed constant, while the stories evolved to fit the changing circumstances of the group. They showed that the transformation of

US nursing into a graduate occupation at that time was being accompanied by a reworking of the stories told about Florence Nightingale. The 'Lady of the Lamp', mopping the brows of fevered soldiers in the Crimean War (1853–56), was giving way to an emphasis on her career as a public health reformer and statistician. She was, for example, the first woman to be elected as a Fellow of the Royal Statistical Society and to be awarded the Order of Merit, the UK's highest honour for services to science, culture and arts. The continuity of the profession was marked by the continuity of references to its iconic heroine: its evolution, in response to changes in medical technology, disease patterns and the division of labour, was marked by a shift that emphasised different aspects of the historical record of Miss Nightingale's career. Nurses were still her successors, even if they were less engaged in hands-on care.

This is not the only use made of Florence Nightingale. If you look at the 19th-century images, you can see religious elements – a famous picture in the National Portrait Gallery is lit almost as if it were a nativity scene. It projects a view of nursing as a calling rather than a skilled trade. The emphasis on Miss Nightingale focuses attention on her elite background at the expense of the ordinary nurses who worked with her in the Crimea. Their stories are almost completely lost. She is an idealised 19th-century woman. If you know a little more about the history of the Crimean War, you might also ask why she was given such high-profile recognition. This was a rather pointless conflict arising from the implosion of the Ottoman Empire and the campaigns were badly mismanaged by all the armies involved. Politically inconvenient truths were obscured by the celebration of a saintly figure.

This version of nursing persists in many lay circles and is responsible for recurrent dismissals of the intellectual demands made on modern nurses. Journalists and politicians perpetuate the belief that any nice, middle-class, girl, however dim, who cares enough, can be a nurse. It was never an accurate description of the nursing workforce beyond a few elite hospitals. As UK nursing developed in the late 19th century, it recruited the daughters of small farmers and lower-middle class or 'respectable working class' families (Dingwall et al., 1988). It also drew in a lot of young migrant women from rural Ireland and, after World War II, from the Caribbean and other former colonies. These women often suffered poor treatment and discrimination within the profession.

When the UK health system began to adjust to its place in a more diverse society, Florence Nightingale began to seem a less unifying figure. Could the white daughter of a well-off family really be an icon for a profession that was increasingly challenged to re-examine its treatment of members from black and minority ethnic (BAME) backgrounds? The search for a BAME ancestor figure eventually settled on a Jamaican-born woman called Mary Seacole (1805–1881), who was a contemporary of Florence Nightingale and also worked in the Crimea. Mrs Seacole wrote an autobiography which was first published in 1857 (Seacole, 2005). This memoir was written as part of a fund-raising campaign, when she was bankrupt, and should be read in that context. However, its narrative of her Crimean experiences is confirmed in most key respects by other sources.

By her own account, Mrs Seacole travelled to England early in 1854 to pursue investments that she had made in gold mining shares, using the profits from earlier grocery and hospitality businesses in Jamaica and Panama. The shares proved to be worthless and she came up with the idea of going to the Crimea, where some of the regiments she had traded with in Jamaica were now fighting. Initially, it seems that she did try to go in some kind of nursing capacity, but the two parties recruited to work under Miss Nightingale's supervision had already left. The relevant government departments were not interested in recruiting more women. (Her CV would probably not have qualified her anyway because most of those who had been employed came from the London hospitals where nursing reform was already under way.) She came up with a different project, of establishing a 'British Hotel' where officers could convalesce. This enterprise would also sell provisions, including home remedies. She went to the Crimea with her business partner at the end of 1854, after the bloodiest part of the campaign. In the event, she never provided accommodation: contemporary accounts describe the business as a combination between a tavern, a café and a grocery store, housed in a couple of iron huts, much like today's shipping containers. When there was a battle, she went off to sell wine and sandwiches to the spectators. It may seem odd today, but battles at this period were spectator sports – fashionable Washington society drove out to watch the early battles of the American Civil War, for example. After the battles she helped to search for wounded or dying soldiers. This was a traditional role for women who accompanied regiments to war, whether as wives, camp-followers or, in this case, traders.

Mrs Seacole's memoir forms the main basis of her transformation into an icon of nursing since the 1980s. She is also the subject of many artefacts. University buildings, scholarships and hospital wards have been named for her. Nursing textbooks celebrate her alongside Florence Nightingale. The study of her life and work has been inserted into the National Curriculum used in English secondary schools. Historic markers have been placed on buildings in London where she lived, and a statue was erected in 2016. Her life has been featured in television programmes for a variety of audiences. The popular *Horrible Histories* series was forced to delete a cartoon sequence showing a fight between Mary Seacole and Florence Nightingale that implied that Miss Nightingale was a racist who had stolen credit for the foundation of the nursing profession.

CRITICAL THINKING EXERCISE

Repeat the previous activity identifying some memorabilia of Mary Seacole buildings, plaques, statues and so on.

Compare and contrast the contemporary images of Mary Seacole with those of Florence Nightingale (see Figures 8.1 and 8.2).

Both of these images are from widely-circulating 19th-century print media. Look at the way in which the scenes are lit and labelled ('Vivandière' is French for a woman who followed the army to sell provisions to the soldiers). How are the characters dressed? How are they interacting with each other? What can you see in the backgrounds?

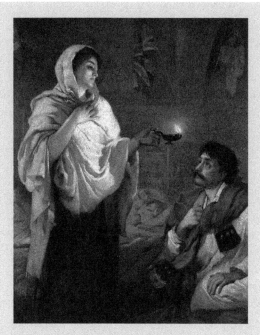

Figure 8.1   Miss Nightingale at Scutari, 1854

Credit: Henrietta Rae, 1891; Wellcome Collection Creative Commons Licence CC-BY

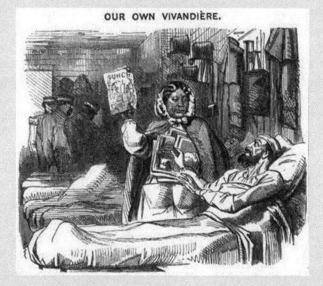

Figure 8.2   Mrs Seacole in the satirical magazine *Punch* distributing copies to wounded soldiers, 1857

The point of this information is that, unfortunately, there is really nothing in the historical record to justify any of this. This has been dissected in detail by Lynn McDonald (2014), a Canadian sociologist, but here are two brief examples.

First, Mrs Seacole never describes herself as a nurse in the sense of someone who is a member of a distinctive occupation associated with the care of sick or injured people in an institutional environment. She writes about herself as a 'doctress, nurse and mother', but her references to nursing are linked to domestic settings, where most 19th-century women would have provided care of sick family members. 'Doctress' seems to have been a term used by traditional healers in Jamaica at that time and has no particular implications of a claim to practise medicine in the modern sense. She never contributed to the 'new profession for women' envisaged by Florence Nightingale.

Second, Mrs Seacole underlines the differences between her role and that of Miss Nightingale. She describes one friendly encounter where Miss Nightingale found her a bed for the night despite the overcrowding in the hospital and she writes acutely about the conditions there and the stress on the nurses. Alexis Soyer, the Jamie Oliver of his day, who knew both women, records carrying mutual good wishes between them (Soyer 1857: 433-6). Mrs Seacole also underlined the difference between her frosty reception from Selina Bracebridge, Miss Nightingale's deputy, which may have had a racist element, and the warmth of Miss Nightingale herself. This is consistent with other evidence of Miss Nightingale's principles: in her first job, as superintendent of a nursing home for women, she clashed sharply with the board over their desire to exclude Catholic and Jewish women. Miss Nightingale and Mrs Seacole were not competitors for credit because they were doing different things.

How, then, did Mrs Seacole come to be an icon? She was a minor celebrity in her own day, popular with the officers who were her customers and friendly with William Russell, the *Times* journalist who covered the war and promoted her cause when she fell into poverty. She did not particularly identify as black: her own background was mixed-heritage and, in her book, she is frequently critical of her black servants' lack of enterprise and work ethic. Why would the UK nursing profession choose to make this woman into a heroine during the 1990s? How can we explain this? What signal is being sent by attaching her name to various kinds of artefact? Why at that time, more than a hundred years after her death in relative obscurity? Why not choose some of the other available black women nurses? Lynn McDonald (2019) offers the example of Kofoworola Abeni Pratt (c.1910/1915–1992), who is believed to have been the first black nurse to work in the British NHS, was active in anti-colonial movements, and played a central role in the decolonisation of Nigerian nursing. She was prominent in international nursing organisations, honoured by the Red Cross and awarded an honorary fellowship by the Royal College of Nursing. We will leave this question with you. What do the Seacole artefacts say about nursing and the place of BAME women compared with, say, the example of Mrs Pratt? Why would she not be such an acceptable icon? Why would it be more difficult for her to be the public face of the profession and enlist public support for its members and their work?

———————— FREEING OUR IMAGINATION ————————

Compare these widely-reproduced images of Mary Seacole and Kofoworola Abeni Pratt. Figures 8.3 and 8.4 are images of possible pioneer black nurses. Which one would you rather be represented by? Why?

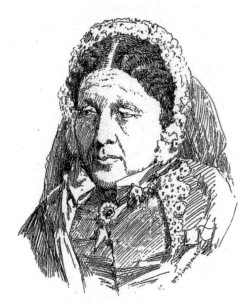

Figure 8.3   Mary Seacole around 1855

Credit: William Simpson

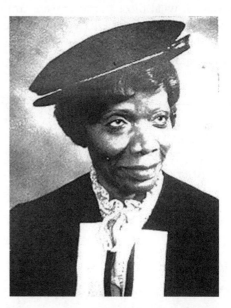

Figure 8.4   Kofoworola Abeni Pratt, 1979

Credit: Vantage Publishers, Ibadan

Can you analyse and comment on the differences? Think about whether you would rather be represented by a well-meaning, middle-aged woman or by an educated professional?

———————————————————————————————————————

This section has given you some idea of the wide range of materials that could be used in a qualitative research project. They can help you to understand more about your profession and the places where you work, as well as thinking about your relationships with patients. Do they see you as Florence Nightingale or Mary Seacole? Which version of Florence Nightingale or Mary Seacole would you like to be seen as? What other images could you construct? How could you do that?

In this section, we have also underlined another principle of qualitative research, namely that we try to be even-handed in our scepticism. This is sometimes called the principle of *symmetry*, that we do not treat heroes and villains in different ways but try to see them within the same framework. If we can try to understand Florence Nightingale through artefacts, we can also understand Mary Seacole in the same way. If we ask how each became an icon, we should ask the same questions about the choices that were made and the influences that were brought to bear in shaping historical evidence to create a story that was fit for a particular purpose within a particular time and place. We can ask what those purposes were and what they say about the people who created them and became advocates for them. We can also ask about their audiences. Who is being encouraged to think what about the profession – or about any other organisation that is trying to convince the people that it deals with that it is doing a good job and is worth supporting?

VIDEO SUPPORT

A useful history of analysing documents is that of Graham Gibbs who gives a lecture on *Documents in Social Research: Part 1 of 2 on Documents and Diaries* and *Document Analysis: A How to Guide* by Jennifer Blank. You can access these videos by visiting this book's online resources: https://study.sagepub.com/dingwallandstaniland.

Key Point

Three suggested stages for analysis are:

- *Preparation* –identify which materials are suitable and relevant for analysis.
- *Review* – study the material, taking note of relevant information and listing follow-up questions for the stakeholders.
- *Organise data* – review notes with stakeholders, organise requirements and seek answers to follow-up questions.

THE SOCIAL CONSTRUCTION OF ORGANISATIONAL STATISTICS

One of the things you might notice about modern health care is the obsession with numbers. Everything must be measured so that it can be counted and managed. What is often forgotten is that all quantitative data starts from qualitative judgements or processes. This does not mean that it is useless or misleading. It can be very valuable to have a common currency that easily allows things to be ranked and compared. This is, after all, how money developed and drove out barter as a basis for economic life. When you are working, you get paid in cash, or in equivalent credit in your bank account, not in loaves of bread, bunches of carrots or rolls of toilet paper. You don't go to the bakers with a pack of sausages to exchange for a pack of buns. Imagine supermarket shopping if you had to push round a trolley full of things you had brought with you to exchange for the things you wanted to take away, and haggle at the checkout about whether they added up to the same value!

It is the same in hospital. When you say that a patient has a temperature of 38°C, everyone knows exactly what you mean, and what the implications might be. If you just said 'This patient seems a bit hot to me', your colleagues will be much less certain. Are your standards of what counts as 'a bit hot' the same as theirs? Perhaps some of them have worked in wards where infections are rare, so 'a bit hot' is not very significant. Others might have more experience of infection and think you are referring to a patient who is about to become very seriously ill. Our first case study will look at these sorts of measurements. Our second case study will look at the use of numbers to compare organisations, or, indeed, whole countries, to understand their performance. You might have filled in a national student satisfaction survey about your course. Suppose 95 per cent of the students on your course are satisfied or very satisfied but the course in the next city only scores 90 per cent, what is this really telling us? Maybe you have nicer teachers who are generous with their marks, while the other course has stern teachers who demand higher standards from their students. Which is the 'better' course?

CASE STUDY SCENARIO 1

When you put a digital probe into a patient's ear to measure their temperature, you probably do not think about the fact that you are using a piece of technology with nearly two thousand years of history behind it. Until the early 18th century, however, each inventor's thermometer was unique so their readings could not be compared. They were not much better than the descriptions we mentioned earlier. This was recognised as a problem for the practice of science and several scales were proposed between 1701 and 1750. Three of these competed for adoption by the scientific community: those devised by Daniel Gabriel Fahrenheit, Anders Celsius, and René Antoine Ferchault de Réaumur. The story of this competition is partly about national pride and partly about technical superiority. The Réaumur scale, which had 80 points between the freezing and boiling points of water, found little favour outside France and its instruments were less reliable. The Celsius scale had 100 measurement points, which made it consistent with the later development of the metric system of measurement. This was adopted by the Revolutionary Government in France and imposed across Continental Europe as a result of the victories of the Napoleonic armies. The French continued to be the principal guardians of the metric system, including the Celsius scale, until 1875, when this was taken over by an international organisation.

Fahrenheit lived much of his life in the Netherlands and was better connected with Britain. He invented 'mercury in glass' thermometers, which came to

(*Continued*)

(Continued)

dominate the world market until very recently; NHS hospitals began to phase them out during the 1990s and they were banned for home use in 2009. Fahrenheit's scale was preferred throughout the English-speaking world. If you go to the USA, you will still find public weather forecasts that use this scale. While most US hospitals work in Celsius, their nurses have to deal with patients who think in Fahrenheit!

There is, of course, a lot more to be said about this history, but this should be enough to show that, behind every simple number on a display or read-out, there is a long history of social actions. With the most successful technologies, these are made invisible by a process called *black-boxing* – the history is wrapped up in a piece of kit that everyone uses and which produces the same numbers. Mercury thermometers were phased out mainly because of the risks of breakage and the release of a toxic element. However, they were also hard to read with great precision. There was always an element of judgement in whether they had been in the patient's mouth for long enough and some variation in where the user thought the mercury had reached on the scale. Digital thermometers time themselves and give a firm number. Data are produced quickly, in a standard form. You do not need to open the box and understand what is happening inside or how it got to be that way – which is very convenient for most everyday purposes.

Definition

A **black box** is an artefact that receives inputs and produces outputs without the internal processes being visible to the ordinary user.

Black-boxing can, though, be dangerous if it is used uncritically. Recall that RD was almost a victim of this when he was hospitalised some years ago for septic shock. He was connected to a digital blood pressure monitor, which appeared to show that he was not responding to infusions intended to revive his blood pressure. The ward team of nurses and junior doctors were increasingly concerned about this and eventually summoned the night duty consultant. He took RD's pulse manually and found that its strength was inconsistent with the monitor reading. An old-fashioned mercury sphygmomanometer was located, which showed that his blood pressure was satisfactory. The digital monitor was faulty, but everyone on the ward had assumed that it must be correct. You might see this as raising a set of qualitative research questions about the role of knowledge and experience. Would the younger generation of staff on the ward have the same ability to contrast a manual pulse with a machine reading and question the machine?

The standardisation of measurements is fundamental to modern science and medicine. It allows people to exchange information freely on a global basis and greatly simplifies practice. However, it always rests on a social agreement that we are all going to measure this thing in this way by reference to this scale. In an ideal world, we will make that measurement by all using the same tool, the same black box. As a project, then, you could take any of the numbers that you use in your everyday practice and ask how they came to be defined and adopted. Why did one scale win over another? Are there differences between things that can easily be standardised, like temperature and blood pressure, and things where more judgement is required, like mental state assessments? Remember when we asked whether questioning RD about his birthday would be meaningful to someone from a cultural background who did not particularly value birthdays (Bowler, 1993:163). What about metrics that fall in between like the Bristol Stool Scale or the various urine colour charts, where you must make a judgement about the match between a patient's specimen and the chart? How easy is it to agree on this? What happens when different professionals make different judgements? Are there areas where nursing scores compete with medical scores? How are these differences resolved – by a social process of interaction and negotiation, or by reference to a social hierarchy of rank and experience?

CASE STUDY SCENARIO 2

The role of social judgements is even more conspicuous in our other case study, where we look at death registration. This is the basis of one of the oldest official statistics, and supposedly one of the most reliable.

Florence Nightingale used death rates as key evidence for her reforms of hospital practice. It is thought to be one of the hardest indicators of the performance of a hospital or of a health care system – but how is it compiled? In fact, this happens through an elaborate social process, which varies from one country to another. Perhaps comparisons between the performance of different countries are, as we say, comparing apples and oranges – things that cannot really be compared for most purposes because they are so different.

This became a very important political issue during the COVID-19 pandemic. Although most statisticians thought the only reliable data would be the measures of excess deaths produced some months later, many politicians and journalists became obsessed with day-to-day comparisons of league tables that would support claims that one country was doing better (or worse) than another.

(Continued)

(Continued)

Let us start at the beginning. How do we know that someone is dead? Your first answer might be that this is easy – their heart stops beating, their brain shuts down and so on. With modern technology, though, we can keep people's vital functions going for a long time purely with support from the right equipment. If someone's conscious brain is no longer working, it may still be prompting other organs through the autonomous nervous system. You might say, well we will leave this to philosophers and ethicists; nurses are practical people who do not need to worry about such things. On the other hand, if you get the decision wrong, you are killing someone. Are you comfortable with that? Do you want to take a chance on someone prosecuting you for homicide? The practical solution to this problem is to turn to the law.

One of the things that law does is to provide certainty where things are uncertain. If you follow a procedure that is authorised by the law, or by a court, you can feel you have made the right decision. But different countries approach this differently. Many Catholic countries, for example, are uncomfortable with recognising patients in a persistent vegetative state as dead for legal purposes and stopping their life support. Even if you have legal rules, they do not translate themselves into practice. People have to decide what they really mean when applied to a specific case. Your hospital may have a protocol that says there must be a case conference involving particular specialities and professions before turning off life support. A decision to withhold or stop CPR is often a team decision. In neither case, though, will it always be the same individuals in the same room, however much the hospital tries to promote consistency through shared training or a shared culture of decision making. You might say that these are cases at the margin, but they make the argument that death is a social judgement.

Once it is agreed that someone has died, there are then two important actions that need to be taken. First, an official document has to be produced that confirms the fact of death and can be used to authorise funerals, transfers of property, bank accounts and so on. Second, in most developed countries, there is also a need to confirm the cause of death, partly as a measure of the country's general health status and the performance of organisations like hospitals, but also partly to ensure the death has not been caused by a criminal action. Causes of death are usually categorised according to the International Classification of Disease (ICD), which is supposed to ensure that everyone uses the same terms. Confirming the fact of death is generally straightforward in developed countries with civil registration systems, although there are differences of detail in who is responsible for completing the form and in officially validating it for legal purposes. Cause of death is, however, much more problematic.

In the UK, medical death certificates are normally completed by a doctor who has seen the patient within 14 days before death. (In certain circumstances, this responsibility passes to the local coroner as a medico-legal matter.) This doctor records the immediate cause of death and any contributing causes. There is an immediate issue about how that doctor decides which is the main cause and which are secondary causes. If a patient with cancer actually dies after a stroke or a myocardial infarction, which is the main cause? The doctors do not necessarily use the language of the ICD. This certificate is used by next of kin to obtain the official certification of death for legal purposes. The medical details are transcribed onto the official certificate so that the cause of death is part of a public record that anyone can access. The medical certificates are reviewed and coded by lay staff, who have to translate them into ICD categories. In a study of this process in Northern Ireland, Prior (1989) showed how the coders constructed stories about deaths in order to do their work. Although the system is changing with the introduction of a review of medical death certificates by a medical examiner from 2019, the fundamental task of fitting deaths to categories remains unchanged – and a problem that qualitative researchers can investigate.

This problem is accentuated by the variation in how medical information about deaths is dealt with by different countries. In France, for example, information about cause of death is not public – it is treated as strictly confidential, passed to relatives in a sealed envelope, which remains sealed throughout its journey from the local town hall to the central bureau where it is coded and counted. The certifying doctor is not publicly accountable for what they write as cause of death. In the USA, every state has its own procedure – in some, every county does its own thing. Many states resemble the UK system, but others have specialist medical examiners who certify every death, while some leave it to the funeral director to ask the doctors involved and complete the paperwork. Once a year all the numbers are sent to the Centers for Disease Control and Prevention in Atlanta, who add them all up and declare them as national data.

Why does this matter? A large part of the discipline of epidemiology rests on the assumption that death rates are reliable data: the numbers are so large that they swamp any local biases. More thoughtful researchers do recognise some of the problems but are not necessarily interested in investigating them. However, there might be reasons why they matter a lot. The UK NHS, for example, is

(Continued)

(Continued)

thought to perform poorly in the treatment of cancer, as measured by mortality rates, compared with other European countries. However, we also know that doctors in some European countries are very reluctant to tell patients, and their relatives, that they have cancer. This may make it difficult for them to record it as a cause of death, even in a confidential document. Could it be that the 'poor' UK performance is actually the result of greater transparency rather than a real difference in the management of patients? This is a question not a finding, but it is a nice illustration of the importance of understanding the story of statistical measures rather than taking them for granted. Sometimes it is important to open the black box and look inside.

This case study could be repeated for any of the statistics that your hospital, or other employer, produces about its operations. Ask:

- How are the numbers created?
- What instructions are given to people at the front line who fill in forms?
- How are they accountable for what they write? How are the forms processed and coded?
- How do they get to be added up?
- Who uses these numbers? For what purposes?

Some of these stages will now happen inside IT systems. Who wrote the algorithms that check the forms and send them back if they do not seem to be correct? What assumptions about the creation of the numbers are embedded in the algorithms? Where did they come from? How far were the people who completed the forms involved in designing them?

CHAPTER SUMMARY POINTS

The world of documents, and artefacts, is rich and diverse. We have tried to show you the possibilities for working with it, rather than giving detailed instructions. However, you should remember the lessons from previous chapters. If you are looking at a document or an artefact, be as specific as possible about what makes it evidence for your arguments. Focus on details – even the small print or the touch from a painter's finest brush can be important. Ask:

- Who the audience is for these statements?
- What is their author trying to say?
- What are their readers or viewers or listeners actually hearing? Why might these be different? Who gets to decide when intentions and responses differ?
- Who designs systems and who uses them? Are they the same people?

FURTHER READING

If you are interested in the ideas set out in this chapter, these books will help you to take them further:

Prior, L. (2003) *Using Documents in Social Research*. London: Sage.

Emmison, M., Smith, P. and Mayall, M. (2012) *Researching the Visual*. London: Sage.

Banks, M. and Zeitlyn, D. (2015) *Visual Methods in Social Research* (2nd edn). London: Sage.

Kara, H. (2017) *Creative Research Methods in the Social Sciences: A Practical Guide*. Bristol: Policy Press.

Two further examples of research studies relevant to nursing using approaches discussed in this chapter: the first compares the images of pregnancy and childbirth presented to women through ante-natal literature in the UK and Japan; the second looks at how nurses actually complete records in the course of their everyday work:

Dingwall, R., Tanaka, H. and Minamikata, S. (1991) 'Images of parenthood in the United Kingdom and Japan', *Sociology*, 25(3): 423–46. Available at https://doi.org/10.1177/0038038591025003005 (accessed 29/2/20).

Tajabadi, A., Ahmadi, F., Sadooghi Asl, A. and Vaismoradi, M. (2019) 'Unsafe nursing documentation: a qualitative content analysis', *Nursing Ethics*, Online First. Available at https://doi.org/10.1177%2F0969733019871682 (accessed 29/2/20).

See also:

Hills, T., Proto, E., Sgroi, D. and Seresinhe, C.I. (2019) 'Historical analysis of national subjective wellbeing using millions of digitized books,' *Nature Human Behaviour*, 3: 1271–5. Available at https://doi.org/10.1038/s41562-019-0750-z (accessed 29/2/20).

9

What do You do with Your Data?

Learning Outcomes

At the end of this chapter you will be able to:

- Discuss the importance of the organisation and categorisation of data in qualitative research
- Outline the use of paper or electronic databases to cross-reference topic codes
- Identify ways of coding data from literature reviews, reading and fieldwork
- Discuss induction and deduction
- Identify the difference between correlation and causation
- Outline the search for truth
- Recognise, connect and validate conclusions
- Outline internal strategies and fair dealing
- Outline external strategies, triangulation and respondent validation
- Summarise key points within the chapter

Qualitative research is not the only way in which we can learn about the world in which we live. Quite apart from quantitative research, there are also bodies of qualitative work from journalists, documentary film-makers, and creative artists like novelists, playwrights or choreographers, that represent and comment on everyday life, institutions and issues of policy and politics. Many of these products are more vivid and immediately engaging than qualitative research reports. What makes qualitative research different? Why might we sometimes prefer it to other sources of information?

The answer to these questions does not lie in the specific methods used by qualitative researchers. As we pointed out in Chapter 1, anybody who is trying to solve a problem is likely to use some of them. A training in qualitative research may help you to use these methods in a more sophisticated and reflective way – but it is a difference of kind rather than degree. Journalists also ask questions and carry out observations: the *Guardian* journalist, Polly Toynbee (2003), for example, took several minimum-wage jobs in order to learn more about the lives of the working poor. The television schedules are overrun with documentary series about life in hospitals. Method actors may spend time living in a role before playing it: Daniel Day-Lewis spent eight weeks in a cerebral palsy clinic in Dublin before filming *My Left Foot* (1989). Artists, musicians and choreographers have long taken everyday life as a source of inspiration, transforming naturally-occurring scenes, soundscapes or movements into works that both reproduce and comment on their properties.

Most of our rivals are interested in the specific stories that they can create from their inquiries. These will be presented in dramatic formats which are intended to engage the emotions of their audiences. This often involves simplification and a focus on extreme events. Qualitative researchers may be equally passionate about what they hope to achieve through their work. They are, though, more interested in their data as a case study that throws light on how people, organisations and societies go about everyday life. What can we learn from this research site about some general issue? Their reports contribute to understanding complex systems and interactions rather than provoking a generalised sense of concern or outrage. They may, of course, uncover serious personal or social troubles that should move people to action. However, this action is, at least ideally, based on a deeper understanding of the complexity of the issues involved and of the points of leverage that are likely to be effective.

The big difference between qualitative research and its rivals, then, is its approach to analysis. If you are still with us, you might be sitting here now overwhelmed with field notes, reflective diaries, interview transcripts, audio or video recordings, copies of key documents, and wondering what you do with them. This is the really difficult bit. You will find any number of qualitative research reports that talk about themes 'emerging' from the data. You may ask why this mysterious process is not happening for you. The reason is that it does not really work like that at all. Themes have to be extracted, which requires a systematic process of looking very closely at your data, testing the conclusions that you draw from it, and then linking these to a wider body of scientific literature. This process takes us back to issues that we first looked at in Chapters 2, 3 and 4 so you might like to re-read those before going further.

GETTING ORGANISED

———————————— VIDEO SUPPORT ————————————

Dr John Schulz gives detailed comprehensive step-by-step guidance on how to analyse qualitative interviews in his video *Analysing Your Interviews*, which you can use as an introduction or revision. You can access the video by visiting this book's online resources: https://study.sagepub.com/dingwallandstaniland.

The first thing you need to do with your data is to organise it so you can easily work with it, move through it, and find the passages that you want to look at in more detail. How you do this is very much a matter of personal preference. It depends on how comfortable you are with working on screen as opposed to working with paper. For most student projects up to PhD scale, paper is often better – remember people have been using it for more than two thousand years so it is a highly sophisticated technology! On the other hand, it may not be quite as portable, and it does have some costs in printing and in environmental impact. We generally prefer working with paper on smaller projects, but perhaps that is just because neither of us are digital natives!

If you want to use paper, the first thing to do is to get all your data into a standard format on paper that is the same size with text that has similar layout and margins that are wide enough to make notes in. If you are dealing with copies of documents, you may not be able to do this exactly, but do the best you can. We find it useful to keep the data in one or more ring binders so that sheets are less likely to get muddled or lost, but you may prefer card folders or treasury tags through the page corners. We also make at least two copies – one will be kept clean so that we can refer to it without any of the marks that we are about to add.

Make sure that each page is numbered. You can either do this consecutively or devise a code that identifies a date, a setting or an interview – 020219/1, Ward1/01, Interview 15/01, for example. The system does not matter: the important thing is that each page has a unique number so that you can easily find it again – and if you take it out of your file, you can put it back in the same place. These unique numbers will be one part of the coding system, which will function like an index to the data. You can go quickly from the theme or topic code to the places where you have relevant material. If you have some knowledge of databases, you can set one up that cross-references your topic codes against the locations where they occur so you can assign topic codes to each page and then get a print-out of the locations you need to go back to for each topic. Don't worry if you don't have that skill, or can't borrow it from someone else, because many small projects work perfectly well by just having a sheet for each topic and writing the location codes onto that.

If you keep your data in an electronic format, the principles are the same. However, you can make use of specialist software like NVivo or ATLAS.ti to help you with indexing and retrieval. There are quite a number of CAQDAS (Computer Assisted Qualitative Data Analysis Software) packages on the market. Your university may have licences for one or two in particular, but you can find independent advice at www.surrey.ac.uk/computer-assisted-qualitative-data-analysis (accessed 29/2/20). More detailed help on using software can also be found in Silver and Lewins (2014). Opinions are rather divided on how useful these packages are for small projects. As we keep saying, your resources are limited, and you need to work efficiently. Is it profitable to invest time in learning how to use these tools and formatting your data to fit them? If you were working on a big project with a team of researchers, then we would certainly recommend using a CAQDAS package. They do make it easier to handle a large body of data with several people working on it at the same time. We would always encourage you to take up any training opportunities that your university may offer so that you know what your options are. However, you must also understand that they will not do the work of analysis for you, any more than a statistics package will in quantitative research. You still have to ask the right questions and code the material in the right way. In a large data set, the software may make it easier to check out some of your hunches – do code 101 and code 142 really tend to occur in the same places at the same times? They are also flexible in terms of breaking down categories – Code 82 has 600 entries so I want to look at it again and see whether I can find more specific sub-topics under this heading – or merging them – Code 35 and Code 90 seem to be capturing the same things so we can put them together.

CODING THE DATA

Now that you have your data organised, the next task is to draw up a coding sheet, which you will use to create an index. This means that you must make some decisions about what you want to get out of the data. In some ways, this is the hardest bit of the whole process. While you can add codes as you go through your data, you do not want to create a lot of work for yourself in going back to review material that you have already been through. It is much more efficient to spend time at the beginning thinking about what you want to get out of the data, even if this means creating some codes that you do not use later when you come to write up your dissertation.

> ## Key Point
>
> Codes come from three sources:
>
> - *Your literature review* – what questions did you identify? What evidence will be relevant to those questions?
> - *Your wider reading* – in what ways might your case study be similar to, or different from, comparable cases elsewhere?
> - *Your fieldwork* – when did somebody say or do something that surprised you, or the other people around them?

In a student project, you do not need many codes. RD's child protection study had nearly 200, but it was based on four years' fieldwork by three people in organisations serving law, social work and health care. A more recent project on learned societies had about 20 codes for 15 interviews. The number of codes would not have increased significantly with a greater number of interviews because the research was focused on a specific problem, much like most student projects. If you do develop a lot of codes, you may find it helpful to group them under higher-level categories, so it is easier to identify them as you go through the data. We shall refer to these higher-level categories as themes and the codes as relating to topics within those themes. Where appropriate, the topic codes should be *axial* – this means that they should have a specific direction. You would not, for example, have a code for 'comments about hospital management' but two codes for 'positive comments…' and 'negative comments…'.

────────────────── **VIDEO SUPPORT** ──────────────────

How to Know You Are Coding Correctly: Qualitative Research Methods has some useful tips on coding, and *How to Code a Document and Create Themes* is one example of how to do coding. You can access these videos by visiting this book's online resources: https://study.sagepub.com/dingwallandstaniland.

──

Let us go back to the project we designed in Chapter 3 and think about what a coding scheme could look like. We were asking whether poor oral care on a ward reflected a problem with the protocol or with the nurses. Suppose you have decided to focus on the ward and the implementation of the protocol, rather than the history of the protocol itself. Your data came partly from participant observation and partly from interviews. This would allow you to identify two themes: the protocol and the practice. The first of these might cover topics like knowledge of the protocol, access to the protocol, and assessments of the relevance and value of the protocol. The second might cover topics like who actually does oral care, when it takes place, and what its priority is among other tasks on the ward. It is most helpful if you can come up with one- or two-word descriptions of the topics because it will be easier to use your coding scheme if it fits onto a single page. You could end up with something that looks like the example in Figure 9.1 – note particularly how we have set up axial codes.

> In **axial coding**, you are using *your concepts and categories* while re-reading the text to confirm that your concepts and categories accurately represent interview responses and to start exploring how your concepts and categories are related.

Definition

Protocol	Nurses
1. Knowledge	1. Care by students
2. Access – when	2. Care by agency staff
3. Access – how	3. Care by healthcare assistants
4. Positive value	4. Care by registered nurses
5. Negative value	5. Care by visitors
6. To be followed	6. Care early in shift
7. A basis for professional judgement	7. Care late in shift
	8. Care abandoned for other task
	9. Other task abandoned for care
	10. Criticism of care
	11. Praise for care

Figure 9.1   Model coding sheet

CRITICAL THINKING EXERCISE

Would you make the code for 'knowledge' of the protocol axial? Would this scheme allow us to distinguish people who know what the protocol says, even if they do not need to look it up all the time, from people who have never heard of it? Is there another category – of people who know the protocol exists but have never looked at it, or been taught to use it, and just do oral care in the same way as everyone else?

Should the axial codes for 'criticism' and 'praise' of care be broken down at this stage so you know whether these judgements are being expressed by other nurses, by patients or by visitors? Is this something you might consider doing at a later point?

Once you have a coding sheet, you should now begin to go through your data and mark the passages that correspond to the codes. At the same time, you should have another sheet for each code on which you should list the locations at which each code occurs. In practice, there are several different ways in which you can do this, which we shall discuss shortly.

Whatever you do, there are three important things you are trying to achieve:

1   You are going to read every line of your data very carefully because you have to decide which code, if any, is relevant. If there isn't a relevant code, should you add one? Perhaps some of your field notes or transcripts really are just filler, the sort of sociable talk that you might do at the beginning or end of an interview to establish or conclude a relationship. You probably do not need a code for questions about the best corridor to walk down to find the hospital bus stops, for example.

2   You are going to think about what specifically makes a passage in your data evidence for a topic. You might have written that a visitor seemed angry about the neglect of a patient. However, that is just your impression and it is not very valuable as evidence. If you had written, 'The visitor said it was shocking how poor the oral care was now compared with her days as a nurse. She said she really wanted to complain to the sister, but she thought that would probably mean her relative just received worse treatment', then you can make a specific link between the visitor's actual words, your interpretation and your decision to code this as 'Criticism of care'.

3   You are going to start breaking up the linear flow of your notes and interviews in favour of making collections of data extracts that relate to specific issues. Your data are being sliced up in a radically different way, so you are breaking with one kind of story in order to tell another.

> ## REFLECT ON PRACTICE
>
> Would a piece of data like this suggest you might want to add a code so you could distinguish between 'expert' visitors with some ability to make a technical judgement on the quality of care and 'naïve' visitors who could only judge whether the staff seemed to be nice while they were around?

You do not want to do this completely. When you come to write your dissertation, you may want to bring data extracts back together in order to construct a case history and to tell an exemplary story – but for now that is not your focus.

HOW DO WE DO THIS?

First, we prepare a set of sheets for the topic codes. Unless you have a lot of data, you probably don't need a sheet for each code. Where we have axial codes like Nurses 10 and 11 above, we would probably have one sheet and draw a line across the middle. Similarly, with Nurses 1 to 5, we might consider having one sheet with five sections. The advantage of the location codes is that they don't take up a lot of space. We then look at the first page. Our personal preference is to use the margins to draw lines that mark the approximate boundaries of topics and to write the topic number beside them. Some people underline blocks of text, possibly with different coloured pens, or use different coloured highlighters. We don't find these work quite as well because blocks of text can have multiple codes and block boundaries may be different for different topics. People who like to work on screen may create folders for each topic and copy relevant text blocks into the folder. The resulting collections may be easy to work with but there is some risk of losing track of their original locations and context. If you have used a CAQDAS package, this will usually tag the text so you can create collections as you need them and move from an extract back to the original. This makes it easier to recover the context and reconsider the boundaries you have marked, or the extent to which the data that interest you have been created by a response to someone else's actions (including yours!).

When you have completed this process, you will have a set of marked field notes where every line has been considered for its possible topic codes and a set of topic code sheets, computer folders or tags that, in principle, list all the locations at which those topics occur. At this stage, some qualitative researchers, especially from disciplines with more quantitative traditions, suggest that you get someone else to code the data independently and measure the correlation between your coding decisions. Technically, this is a version of *inter-rater reliability*, which is commonly used in certain kinds of psychometric tests.

———————————— **VIDEO SUPPORT** ————————————

It may be useful at this stage to look again at how reliability and validity are achieved in qualitative research. Dr Jurek Kriukow explains this in *Validity and Reliability in Qualitative Research (6 Strategies to Increase Validity)*. You can access the video by visiting this book's online resources: https://study.sagepub.com/dingwallandstaniland.

If you choose to do this, you can, although it will depend on finding a willing associate and having the time to do it. We are not sure that it adds much value to a typical student project. RD and his colleagues did do a certain amount of double reading on the child protection project, but that was mainly because they were concerned to be reasonably consistent between team members and to ensure that they did not miss anything important in over 4,000 pages of data.

Key Point

Remember, the main purpose of the coding is to create an *index for you to use* rather than to count the entries under particular topics and to make quantitative claims about them.

You will establish the reliability and validity of your analysis through its rigour, not from the extent to which someone else happens to agree with your coding decisions. So it is important to remember to keep notes about your coding, as you will need to explain this in your dissertation.

ANALYSING THE DATA

In this section, we are going to return to the discussion of induction and deduction that we began in Chapter 2. You may find it helpful to look at that again, because we are now going to get more technical about the processes involved.

———————————— **VIDEO SUPPORT** ————————————

For your revision, the short video *Inductive Analysis for Analyzing Data* by Andrew Johnson simply explains the process of induction. You can access the video by visiting this book's online resources: https://study.sagepub.com/dingwallandstaniland.

Your next step is to look at the collections of data you have assembled under each of your codes; of course you are only going to do this one code at a time to start with, except where you have created axial codes when you will probably want to be able to compare them. You are going to try to produce a more general and abstract statement of the features of that code. This will take you from specific instances to something that can apply across all, or most of them, and can be transferred to settings that you have not yet seen. The basic logic of this process was set out by the British philosopher John Stuart Mill in *A System of Logic*, first published in 1843. He identified four techniques, which can be combined in five ways:

1   *The method of agreement* – if you have two or more data extracts that have only one feature in common, then that feature is the key to putting them together in a more general way. For example, if you found that you had two observations of poor oral hygiene and both patients had had their care from health care assistants, you could conclude that health care assistants deliver a low quality of oral care. In practice, you would not draw such a strong conclusion from just two observations, but it would be a basis for going through the rest of the data in a process of *constant comparison* to see whether you could make this a generalisation.

2   *The method of difference* – if you have two or more data extracts that are similar in every feature, except for one, then that feature is the basis of the differences between them. For example, if all your poor oral hygiene was performed by health care assistants, except for that by one individual, then you ask what was special about that person. You might find that they were actually a nurse trained outside the UK who was not yet licensed to practice in that role. This would allow you to strengthen your conclusion about the limitations of health care assistants in delivering oral care. In qualitative research, we call this *deviant case analysis*. It is a very important part of validating your conclusions because it shows that you have not just cherry-picked the data that suit the story you wanted to tell at the beginning. You have systematically looked for the cases that do not fit your emerging theoretical framework and developed the framework to accommodate them.

3   *The joint method of agreement and difference* – this combines the two previous techniques. If you have two or more data extracts that share a common feature, and others in which it is absent, then you can claim that this feature plays an important part in your explanations of your find-ings. In the example we have been working with, you can combine the findings about who delivers oral care in order to narrow the focus to health care assistants with a particular social or educational background rather than the problem arising with all health care assistants.

4   *The method of residues* – this works by subtracting the effects of the general statements you have already developed from the case you are looking at and then asking what is left over. For exam-ple, you have concluded that the problem of poor oral care is linked to health care assistants with a particular social and educational background. However, the hospital management now decide to merge two wards, and the pool of health care assistants changes. Some of the original staff remain and continue their previous practice, while the newcomers deliver better care. You can now conclude that the quality of work is not just a product of the assistants' background but is also related to their previous experience – here you might be led to look at the quality of supervision and standards set by the ward leadership.

5   *The method of concomitant variation* – this says that if one thing varies at the same time as another, there is some sort of linkage between them. Suppose, for example, you find that health care assistants deliver better oral care on some shifts than others. You look more closely and discover that those shifts are supervised by a particular ward sister or charge nurse. You can then conclude that quality of supervision may override other limitations in training or experience. With this method, though, you do need to be careful not to confuse *correlation* and *causation*. We shall say more about this shortly.

Key Point

We should stress that we have nothing against health care assistants and the valuable work that they do. We are simply demonstrating how to think your way through the analysis of your data. This is not based on any of our own research and we have no particular reason to think that there is a problem with the care delivered by health care assistants within the scope of their practice.

If you go further in social science, you will discover that some of John Stuart Mill's methods are not quite as straightforward as they might seem when you first meet them. They are, though, still a useful place to start from and the foundation of a great deal of contemporary thinking about scientific method.

DIFFERENCES BETWEEN CORRELATION AND CAUSATION

The difference between correlation and causation is particularly tricky and worth some further comment. You may have come across this in quantitative methods courses, but it is also a problem for qualitative researchers. Just because two things happen at the same time, or in sequence – *correlation* – does not mean that one *causes* the other (or vice versa). If the sun rises at 07.00 hrs and your alarm clock goes off at 07.05 hrs, this does not mean that the sunrise has triggered the alarm.

———————————————— VIDEO SUPPORT ————————————————

In a Wireless Philosophy video *Critical Thinking – Fundamentals: Correlation and Causation*, Paul Henne (Duke University) explains the difference between correlation and causation. You can access the video by visiting this book's online resources: https://study.sagepub.com/dingwallandstaniland.

The classic statement about causation comes from the 18th-century Scottish philosopher, David Hume. A causal relationship must have three elements:

- *Contiguity in time and space* – this does not necessarily mean that two observations are right next to each other, in either time or space, but that a chain of adjacent events can be described that links them. A traffic accident may cause a crisis in a major trauma centre, even though the events are many kilometres apart and separated by the time required for patient transport. However, we can specify all the connections in the form of bystander calls, control centre call handlers, first responders, emergency services and so on.
- *Priority in time* – if you are going to be able to say that A caused B, then A must come before B. You can say that flicking a light switch causes the light to come on because the switching takes place before the bulb or LED lights up.
- A ***necessary*** *connection between cause and effect* – this is the most important test. You have to be able to say that A must be followed by B. For electric circuits, this is simple: the current will not flow unless the switch is closed, so flicking the switch must be followed by the light coming on. The light cannot come on unless the switch is closed. However, it is quite difficult to show this in social science because there are so many possible connections. Even this simple example, though, is not quite as tight as it might seem.

SELF-ASSESSMENT ACTIVITY

Will the light *always* come on when you close the switch and complete the electrical circuit? Can you think of any circumstances when it might not?

In the ideal world of physics, electrical circuits do not contain faulty components, loose connections or defective light bulbs. While the light cannot come on unless the switch is closed – a *necessary* connection – a set of other, *sufficient*, conditions must be satisfied if this is actually to happen. In this example, that set might be quite small. In most everyday-life situations, it is quite large.

Human institutions are very complex, constantly changing and full of interactions and feedback loops. This is what makes social science so challenging. There are very few circumstances where it is possible to satisfy Hume's tests completely. It is best to think of them as disciplining principles for your analysis. Can you develop an argument governed by these principles which makes a plausible case for the connections that you have drawn out from your data? Remember what we said earlier about the importance of small gains. How can your research make things better rather than trying to make them perfect?

THE SEARCH FOR 'TRUTH'

Another issue that qualitative researchers sometimes struggle with is that of 'truth'. We have put this word in quotes because it has become increasingly troublesome for social scientists. Let us try to explain why this is the case. It is partly because of a confusion about what it means to say that something is true. We can start with mathematics, where truth is a matter of logical reasoning from a set of *axioms*. These are the founding principles of the system. If you did geometry at school, you might remember Pythagoras' theorem, that the square of the hypotenuse is equal to the sum of the squares of the two other sides. This is true by definition. It cannot be otherwise if you have correctly followed the principles of geometry first laid down by Euclid, an ancient Greek mathematician. This model had a strong influence on 18th- and 19th-century physics and, through this, on other natural sciences. Nature was out there and the challenge to science was to capture its fundamental laws. Early social scientists also tried to copy this model, which had a strict separation between the observer and the observed.

As time went on, though, the idea that every science could look like physics or mathematics became increasingly problematic. Honest observers just saw the world differently. Early psychology, for example, was partly stimulated by the discrepancies between observations of stars made by different observers (Friedman, 1967). They were looking at the same skies but measuring them differently. Which observer was right, and which was wrong? The psychologists found that it was not a question of accuracy or error but of differences in perception. Different professors saw the stars in slightly different ways and trained their staff and students to do the same. This caused problems when they went to another observatory. Most natural sciences have had similar problems at some point – which they often get around by creating *black boxes*, as we discussed in Chapter 8.

Historians, philosophers and social scientists who studied the actual practice of the natural sciences found that they depended on working agreements to a much greater extent than they had recognised. There was an inevitable gap between the material world or the world of nature and the ways it could be studied. What we thought of as scientific truth today was just the best efforts of current scientists, and there was no reason to suppose that it would not be changed by the next generation.

REFLECT ON PRACTICE

Remember the miasmatic theory of disease, which we mentioned in Chapter 2 – the idea that illnesses were caused and transmitted by bad smells, which was displaced during the 19th century by germ theory, the idea that illnesses were caused and transmitted by micro-organisms that could not be seen with the naked eye. The supporters of miasmatic theory, who included Florence Nightingale, until quite late in her life, were not wrong. They had simply adopted the theory that was shared at the time and seemed to be the best available. In fact, some of the public health actions that people derived from the theory, like installing sewerage systems, were quite effective, even if for the 'wrong' reasons.

The idea that scientific truth was a matter of consensus led some writers to argue that it was *just* a matter of consensus. Any view was as good as any other – and might even be better because it was not constrained by the accepted wisdom. This has led to a great deal of conflict among scientists and scholars, which has carried over into social movements like that of people opposed to childhood vaccination.

─────────────── **FREEING OUR IMAGINATION** ───────────────

We think you should approach the questions about truth like this:

1 People act based on their interpretations or perceptions of the world.
2 These perceptions are anchored in particular times, places and standpoints.
3 However, the world has its own existence, independent of our interpretations or perceptions, although we can only know it through these.
4 This means that encounters with the world can challenge or correct our interpretations or perceptions.
5 Scientific research, including social scientific research, always attempts to constrain possible interpretations by reference to the world. The search for truth disciplines our inquiries.

Technically, this position is called *subtle realism*, if you want to search for more commentary on the philosophical and methodological arguments around it.

> **Subtle realists** accept that there is a material world that exists independently of our perceptions – but we can only know this world through our perceptions, which are influenced both by our physical capacities and by our knowledge and experiences in a particular society at a particular time.

Definition

For now, let us just illustrate it with a more concrete example.

There is currently a problem in many developed countries about the declining uptake of childhood vaccination against measles (Reich, 2016). Several factors are involved in this. The most important is certainly the way in which cuts to public health and primary care services have reduced the access of poor and socially marginal groups to vaccination services. Small numbers of children have always missed out on vaccination because of their parents' religious beliefs. This has not been a problem because so many others have been vaccinated that they get protection from the general level of immunity in the community. However, there has been much higher visibility for the resistance from relatively small but articulate groups of educated parents who subscribe to a variety of libertarian or 'alternative' beliefs about the right to reject 'expert' knowledge in favour of their own judgement. Their decisions are based on their own interpretations (Point 1 above), which are a product of theories that are circulating at a particular time in particular places (2). However, this does not eliminate the reality of an entity that scientists have called a 'virus' since the 1930s, which causes an infection that has been labelled 'measles' since the 15th century (3). This virus can, and does, infect unvaccinated children regardless of their parents' beliefs (4). Scientific research now proceeds on the basis that there is a real disease called measles that is caused by a virus. This approximation is better than previous ones. Measles has been known to be caused by an infectious agent in the blood since the mid-18th century, but the nature of such agents was not understood until the identification of bacteria in the mid-19th century. By the early 20th century, scientists recognised that there had to be other agents, smaller than bacteria, but were unable to identify these with the tools available at the time. Social scientists can describe the institutional processes by which scientists came to change their description of measles from a set of signs and symptoms into the product of a specific virus – a *causal* agent. In the process, other diseases that produce childhood fevers and a rash were identified and distinguished. The natural or material world gradually imposed itself on the accounts offered by biomedical scientists (5). In seeing those accounts as the outcome of social processes, however, social science does not invalidate them. It offers something different, which may help to encourage more flexible thinking within the scientific community by recognising the ways in which thought might be constrained by a variety of organisational constraints. Science is about people and their work just as much as it is about what lies at the end of a microscope or inside an Eppendorf tube.

VALIDATING YOUR CONCLUSIONS

If you have worked your way systematically through your data, this should now have been transformed into a collection of more general and abstract statements, each of which summarises a set of data extracts that represent supporting evidence for that statement. As you produce these more general statements, you should also recognise that some of them are connected. In the previous example, we sketched possible connections between quality of care, the backgrounds of the people who were providing it, the nature of the supervision that shaped their work, and the culture of the organisation that defined what was acceptable. In the next chapter, we will look in more detail at how you turn this collection into a written text. Before we do this, though, we just want to say a few words about how you might test your emerging conclusions. What can you do to demonstrate that you have allowed them to be disciplined by the social world that you have studied? There are two main strategies that you can follow: internal strategies and external strategies. They are not mutually exclusive so you can do both, if you have the time and resources. If not, you might try to adopt at least some of these ideas.

Internal strategies

Internal strategies refer to things that you might do within the framework of the data you have already collected. We have already mentioned deviant case analysis: will you be able to show your readers that you have looked carefully through your data for cases that might not fit your argument? This is particularly important if you are working in an area where people have very strong prior views. There is, for example, currently a lot of debate about 'lad culture' among students and how to draw a boundary between 'banter' and 'harassment'. If you were investigating interactions between men and women students, you would want to be careful to show that you had looked at situations where women joined in sexually-oriented talk and behaviour as well as those where they showed they were offended or upset by it.

An extension of this is what Dingwall (1992; Murphy and Dingwall, 2003) has called the principle of *fair dealing*. What made qualitative research different from the rivals we introduced at the beginning of this chapter was its commitment 'to comprehend the perspectives of top dogs, bottom dogs and, indeed, lap dogs' (Dingwall, 1980: 874). Fair dealing involves communicating equal understanding of both the powerful and the powerless in any situation. It is easy – and many researchers have fallen into this trap – to identify with the underdogs in any context and to write a story about heroes and villains. Nursing research often writes about doctors in this way without attempting to understand how doctors come to act in the ways that they do. The same is often true when writing about managers: they are the enemy of the frontline people doing the hard and dirty work. The managers' actions have a rationality and logic, though. They are not setting out to make life difficult for those beneath them. If you don't understand that logic, you cannot hope to change it. In practice, of course, you may not be able to get to observe or interview all the people in management that you might want to – but you can try to show that you have thought about what their perspective might be rather than just assuming that all the stories you have been told about them are true. Fair dealing does not prevent you from making moral judgements about the contributions of different people or groups, but it does insist that you can clearly separate these from your analysis of the contexts within which your findings have been produced.

Another internal procedure that you might consider is to develop your analysis on only one part of your data and then to use the other part to test it. You use inductive reasoning first and then switch to a more deductive approach. You use your initial analysis to make predictions about what is going to happen in the rest of your data, and then look to see whether it does. If the predictions fail, then you need to revise the analysis. There are relatively few examples of this; the best known is probably P.M. Strong's (2001) influential study of clinics for children with developmental problems.

External strategies

If you read further in the literature on qualitative research, you will soon come across the idea of *triangulation* and its extension, *respondent validation*.

—————————————— **VIDEO SUPPORT** ——————————————

Watch *Triangulation of Evidence* for further explanation of this. You can access the video by visiting this book's online resources: https://study.sagepub.com/dingwallandstaniland.

The idea of triangulation comes originally from surveying and navigation. In order to find out the exact location of a geographical feature, like a hilltop or a ship, you measure its relationship to three other points. Your mobile phone does this invisibly, by reference to the direction of transmission towers, when you use an app for navigation. It has been adopted as a metaphor in qualitative research to describe the idea that you might use different methods to look at the same research problem. If they all give you the same answer, then you can have more confidence in your findings. This idea has stimulated a great deal of mixed-method research, which is often claimed to be more valid than investigations that rely on a single method.

CRITICAL THINKING EXERCISE

At first sight, triangulation probably sounds like a good idea. Can you see any problems with it?
  You may want to look at Chapters 6, 7, and 8 again while you think about this.

This claim is not, though, quite as straightforward as it might seem. Why doesn't it always make sense to use different methods to check on each other? There are some important problems with triangulation:

1   *What do you do when the methods do not give you the same answer?* This is a very important methodological problem. Can you use a technique to show something is true, if you cannot use the same technique to show that it is false? Most writing on triangulation assumes that the findings from different methods will more or less agree. However, nothing says they have to. You may have data from observation and interviews. We explained earlier why qualitative researchers thought that observation was the gold standard for their work. If your interview data tell you a different story, which one do you believe? Are you going to discard the findings of the best method by reference to the second best? In practice, as Silverman (2017) has suggested, such discrepancies become the starting point for further analysis. How come the world looks so different between you observing it and the participants talking to you about it? Does it tell you something about the way in which they see you or the way in which they would like to be represented?

In RD's child protection study, for example, he routinely interviewed the directors of various local agencies involved in this work. He would outline some of the emerging findings about the problems that confronted people working directly with these cases. These were often dismissed or played down by these high-level informants. RD came to realise that he was being treated as if he were some kind of journalist and that senior managers were constrained by the nature of their position and institutional context to talk about their agencies in positive ways. They knew the realities of the street as well as he did, but they were expected to talk up the work of their organisation when placed on the record. In the course of trying to understand the discrepancy, RD had learned something about what it meant to be an agency director.

REFLECT ON PRACTICE

Do different methods tell you the same things anyway?

If you look back at the last three chapters, you should recognise that the three main qualitative methods are giving you different pieces of a jigsaw, which is completed by the work of quantitative researchers. *Observation* tells you about the way in which the participants go about creating their everyday world through their interactions with each other in particular contexts. *Interviews* tell you how they create stories, which, they hope, will make sense to you, about how and why the world works in the way that it does. *Documents* tell you how they try to give that world some kind of stability and permanence beyond the moments of interaction that you can observe. Quantitative studies (e.g. counting the cows) give you more precise descriptions of the distributions of people, characteristics or events, and of certain kinds of inputs and outputs. These are very important for many purposes but have their limitations when it comes to understanding the processes that create these distributions or outcomes. If patients from minority backgrounds report more dissatisfaction with their treatment in surveys, for example, does this result from different initial expectations or different interactions with the health workers providing services to them? Mixed-method studies, then, are less about using the methods to check on each other than about assembling a more comprehensive picture by looking at a problem from different angles.

'Respondent validation' refers to the idea that you could validate your findings by taking them back to your informants and asking for their agreement or approval. This has been given a particular boost by the pressure for *patient and public involvement* (PPI) throughout the research process. PPI, and related approaches like action research or participatory action research, can be valuable in promoting the engagement of people who might benefit from the research. The consultative processes involved may alert the researchers to angles and issues that they had not fully considered in planning their work. The level of engagement can mean that the research is more useful in bringing about changes. However, these processes can also create methodological problems. If we emphasise the problems here, it is because you will probably encounter a good deal of advocacy for participative qualitative research methods.

CRITICAL THINKING EXERCISE

If you look back at the discussion of triangulation, can you see any potential methodological problems with PPI?

In fact, many of the same problems arise. What do you do if your informants disagree with you? Does this mean that you have got things wrong – or simply that they do not like the picture you have painted? Disagreement may provoke some new questions but it does not necessarily invalidate your findings. There are two other problems that you might want to think about as well:

- *There is no guarantee that your informants or collaborators will share your motivation and expertise.* Researchers who have tried respondent validation often report a lack of interest among the research participants in looking at their reports, even in a popular or summary form. In some ways, this is not surprising because people move on and the passage of time may make your work seem less immediately relevant. They may also be less interested in the things you are interested in. Remember you are seeing your research site as a case study that you will link to a wider literature. Even if this leads you to quite specific conclusions and recommendations, it is a different way of looking at something that the participants experience as unique. Your *expertise* means you are taking a sideways look at something they are closely engaged in.
- *There is no guarantee that all the people involved in the research will see it the same way.* What do you do if the patients like your depiction of the research site and the nurses hate it? This is something that might suggest some new questions to think about – but should you rewrite your findings? There may also be people who have a relevant view but are not involved. In practice, for example, PPI and similar approaches often exclude the well people who pay for the health and social care system, whether through their taxes or their insurance premiums. This means that it is easy for research to come up with complaints about the limitations of a service for one client group without recognising the choices that are being made within a budget fixed by the willingness of other people to pay for it. It is the same question that we keep asking you about your research: is the service doing the best it can with the resources available, or is it perfect? Having an idea of what perfect would look like is great, but not if it gets in the way of making small practical improvements here and now.

CHAPTER SUMMARY POINTS

This chapter has taken a step-by-step approach to the organisation and categorisation of data in qualitative research. Remember that qualitative data is frequently subjective, rich, and entails in-depth information normally presented in the form of words. Analysing qualitative data necessitates the reading of many transcripts looking for similarities or differences, and then finding themes and emerging categories. The way you do this is a matter of preference: 'cut and pasting' or using of software specifically designed for qualitative data management. Several computer software packages have been developed to mechanise this 'coding' process as well as to search and retrieve data. We revisited induction and deduction and identified the difference between correlation and causation. We also discussed internal and external strategies for validity of data. By now you probably have a lot of notes, jottings and drafts,problem statement, methods, literature review and analysis; in the next chapter we will help you to turn these into a report or dissertation.

FURTHER READING

We suggested two of these books by Howard Becker at the end of Chapter 3 - and we have added a third now that you have made more progress. Becker writes very clearly about sophisticated ideas. Even if you read his work earlier, you will probably find new things to think about if you look at it again.

Becker, H.S. (1998) *Tricks of the Trade: How to Think about your Research while You're Doing it*. Chicago, IL: University of Chicago Press.

Becker, H.S. (2007) *Telling About Society*. Chicago, IL: University of Chicago Press.

Becker, H.S. (2017) *Evidence*. Chicago, IL: University of Chicago Press.

This paper extends the discussion of what counts as quality in qualitative research. It is based on a large historical review of qualitative research methods in health commissioned by a UK health services research agency (Murphy et al., 1998):

Dingwall, R., Murphy, E., Watson, P., Greatbatch, D. and Parker, S. (1998) 'Catching goldfish: quality in qualitative research', *Journal of Health Services Research and Policy*, 3(3): 167–72. Available at https://doi.org/10.1177/135581969800300308 (accessed 29/2/20).

These two papers extend the discussion of CAQDAS and analysis more generally:

O'Kane, P.P., Smith, A. and Lerman, M.P. (2019) 'Building transparency and trust-worthiness in inductive research through Computer-Aided Qualitative Data Analysis Software', *Organizational Research Methods*. Available at https://doi.org/10.1177/1094428119865016 (accessed 29/2/20).

Raskind, I.G., Shelton, R.C., Comeau, D.L., Cooper, H.L.F, Griffith, D.M. and Kegler, M.C. (2019) 'A review of qualitative data analysis practices in health education and health behavior research', *Health Education & Behavior*, 46(1): 32–9.Available at https://doi. org/10.1177/1090198118795019 (accessed 29/2/20).

A useful source on mixed methods is:

Ladner, S. (2019) *Mixed Methods: A Short Guide to Applied Mixed Methods Research*. Sam Ladner (self-published).

This book is also a good example of reading outside the immediate field of health. Sam Ladner is a sociologist who has worked for most of the major US tech companies. This involves collaborations with software designers to understand how their products might be used. Such work is sometimes called UX or User Experience research. It has many parallels with health services research on patient experiences. When Sam writes about the problems of combining qualitative and quantitative methods and of making the case for change, she is addressing problems that you should be familiar with in a different context – which should stimulate you to notice things about patient experience research that you might not otherwise pick up.

10

Writing Your Dissertation

Learning Outcomes

At the end of this chapter you will be able to:

- Identify who you are writing for and what they expect
- Set micro targets for your writing
- Organise the content of your chapters
- Write a conclusion
- Identify good writing in the context of a dissertation

If you have been following us through this book, you should now have accumulated quite a pile of notes, jottings, drafts and so on from the problem statement, literature review, methods statement, data analysis and, we hope, a reference list to date. These materials will form the basis of your dissertation. Some students find it helpful to add up the number of words they have already written in these documents because it reassures them that they have already made a lot of progress towards their dissertation target. When you sit down to write your final version, much of the work should just be polishing these preliminary texts and weaving them together into a coherent whole. You might think this is easier said than done, but our objective in this chapter is to show you how you might do this. We begin by discussing how to think strategically about writing your dissertation.

--- **VIDEO SUPPORT** ---

You may wish to watch *Writing up Qualitative Research* to identify some tips for writing up research findings successfully. You can access the video by visiting this book's online resources: https://study.sagepub.com/dingwallandstaniland

---

WHO ARE YOU WRITING FOR, AND WHAT DO THEY EXPECT?

There are two fundamental questions that you need to answer before you begin any piece of writing: who is going to read it, and what do they expect to read? The commonest mistake that inexperienced writers make is to assume that they are writing to express themselves, and that it does not matter what their readers make of the text. This is fine for certain kinds of creative writing, but it is a disaster for anything that is official, formal or assessed. Just because your writing makes sense to you does not mean that it makes sense to anyone else. You are, however, going to be evaluated on it: if your evaluator cannot understand what you have written, they are not going to give you a high grade. This applies to all your professional writing. Although we are focusing here on your dissertation, you will also be judged throughout your career on the records and reports that you write about your patients or service users, or about the various activities of health service organisations that you are asked to manage or co-ordinate. Writing is one of the most important ways in which you can be an effective advocate for the people in your care. If you start by asking 'Who do I need to convince – and what will it take to convince them?', you will immediately have an advantage.

In the UK, undergraduate and Master's dissertations are often marked by the person who supervised them. These marks will usually be reviewed by another member of the department's academic staff. Some, or all, of these marks will also be reviewed by a member of academic staff in the same discipline from another university. When it comes to PhD theses, the supervisor steps back and the assessment is carried out by a different member of the internal academic staff and an independent external academic. These various processes are intended to achieve the consistent treatment of students who are researching and writing about many different topics. Other countries have different ways of achieving this, but most of the principles here are the same.

PhD students will normally be consulted about likely examiners, and will know who they are, before completing work on their thesis. For undergraduate and Master's dissertations, it may not be as easy to find out who the internal reviewers are likely to be because the department may not decide until after the submission deadline, when it is clear what work needs to be distributed. However, you do have an opportunity to study your supervisor at close quarters and to learn what he or she is looking for in a good dissertation.

Key Point

A good way to start is to look at your supervisor's research profile and publications, in order to identify their approach and areas of interest.

The department will have some standard guidance but, as you have learned, that guidance always has to be interpreted in order to be applied in a specific case. How is your supervisor going to do that? What clues are they giving you when you meet them in supervision sessions? The department will probably expect you, and your supervisor, to keep a joint formal record of these sessions. However, you should think of these meetings as being like fieldwork. Use the skills we discussed in Chapter 6 to make notes of these sessions and review them afterwards. Many supervisors will give you permission to record these sessions. If English is not your first language, you may find this particularly helpful, because you can replay the session and make sure you have picked up all the clues that your supervisor has given you about how to get a good mark. PhD students can still benefit from these tips, but it may be more important for them to look for opportunities to read their examiners' latest writings or to see them in action at a conference or seminar. These are also potential sources of information about what they think good work looks like.

Key Point

Some of our students have downloaded pictures of their supervisor or examiners, printed them off, and pinned them to the wall over their computer as a reminder about the audience for whom they are writing. When the students are stuck over a particular sentence, they look at the picture and ask 'How should I write this for X to understand it?'

Of course, it is also important to look at the formal criteria that your department has laid down for dissertations. We are constantly surprised by how many students do not do this until very late in the process. As we have stressed in earlier chapters, analysing the constraints under which you are working is an essential aspect of using your time and resources efficiently. If your department only asks you to write 10,000 words for a dissertation, it is not a good idea to produce a first draft that is 15,000 words long. You may waste time cutting your text rather than improving it. Equally, if you only write 6,000 words, you will probably not have enough content to be able to get a good grade. However, we recognise that students are different and if you feel that you must write everything down and then edit, then do that.

It is important to know what the target is because this will help you to set micro-targets for each chapter. These will allow you to distribute your effort appropriately. You should also be clear whether your references are included within the overall word limit. In general, we think your first draft should plan to be about 10 per cent under the department's maximum. Why do we say this? Well, most people actually end up writing a little over length, whatever they have started out to do. If you are allowed to write 10,000 words, plan to write 9,000 and find you have written 9,500, you do not have a problem. If you have planned to write 10,000 words and find you have written 10,500, you are going to have to work out how to lose some!

You should also look at the marking criteria that are laid out in your department's guidance. This may either be in a generic student handbook for the course or in a specific handbook for the dissertation element. If this is what your markers are going to look at, then you should use the same information to ask how well you have covered the crucial points.

──────────── **FREEING OUR IMAGINATION** ────────────

Never start your writing with a blank page. If you have been given guidelines for each section/chapter of your dissertation, put these as headings on your blank page and refer to them as you are writing to ensure that you are not diverting from the topic or the guidelines. You may be writing a brilliant paper, but if it doesn't meet the marking criteria it will all be wasted.

Typically, the marking criteria will deal with the structure and organisation of the dissertation; the presentation of existing knowledge and how effectively you have evaluated this; the way you have used that knowledge and what you might have added to it; and your ability to reflect on the whole experience, to draw conclusions from it and to recognise what you might do better in future. Even if the guidance is not explicit about this, your markers will probably have a mental allocation of about 25 per cent of the marks to each of these headings. This tells you that you need to distribute your writing effort in a way that gives each heading a reasonable amount of space. As the minds of markers work, it is generally easier to get the first two-thirds of the mark in each category than the last third; 4 × 17 will easily get you a good upper second-class mark. You can then ask where you might be particularly strong and try to polish your first draft for a 20 or a 21 element that will take you towards a first class.

If you look at the typical headings, you will see that they more or less map on to the material that you have already assembled. The structure and organisation element will relate to the way in which you have set up the research problem, described how you are going to explore it and then done what you promised to do. The presentation and critique of existing knowledge will cover the literature review and the justification for your choice of method. The use of the knowledge and your reflections on it are assessing your data collection and analysis. Your reflections on the experience will be the subject of your conclusion, which we shall say more about in this chapter. Try to make things easy for your marker by thinking about where you can use language from the marking criteria, especially in the conclusion, so they do not have to dig deeply into your text to find things to reward. Remember, your marker may have dozens of dissertations to mark or review – the easier they can find good things in yours, the easier it is to reward them.

──────────── **VIDEO SUPPORT** ────────────

Another useful video to watch which will help you with this is *Writing Tip #3: Writing Qualitative Findings Paragraphs*. You can access the video by visiting this book's online resources: https://study.sagepub.com/dingwallandstaniland.

SETTING MICRO-TARGETS

Once you have identified the audience for your dissertation and the framework within which you need to write it, the next step is to break this down into more specific tasks. What you are trying to do here is to establish how best to allocate your effort within the overall project and to break it into manageable chunks. The latter is particularly important if you are not a confident writer. A 10,000-word dissertation may sound quite intimidating, but if you can see it as just a set of linked 2–3,000 word essays, then you should be faced with a more familiar challenge. Most undergraduates will have experience of writing at this length well before they come to tackle a dissertation. (The same, incidentally, is true for Master's or PhD theses: if you have written a 10,000-word undergraduate dissertation, then these texts are made up of a series of chapters at about that length). Again, be sure to check whether your references are included within the word limit.

Your department may have a preference for chapter titles and themes – your study of the guidance should have told you that. If not, most dissertations have a standard format, which mirrors the order we have worked through in this book: Background and problem statement; Literature review; Justification and description of methods; What you have found; and What you have learned. The main difference between dissertations or theses at different levels is one of scale. An undergraduate dissertation will have shorter chapters and will probably only have one devoted to discussing and analysing the data. MA and PhD theses will have longer chapters with 2–4 of them dealing with the data and analysis. The data chapters will also carry more weight in the assessment because there is a stronger expectation that they will be making an original contribution to knowledge. Undergraduate dissertations are more focused on determining whether you have grasped all the basics involved in doing research. If you can be original as well, that is a bonus. Given this, you should distribute your efforts and available words more or less equally between the chapters. The data chapter may need a little more, and the introduction and conclusion a little less. For a 10,000-word dissertation, you might allocate the space something like this:

1   Background and problem statement, 1,500 words
2   Literature review, 2,500 words
3   Justification and description of methods, 1,500 words
4   Discussion and analysis of data, 3,000 words
5   Conclusion, 1,000 words

This makes 9,500 words, which gives you some margin for slippage. You may very well find that the first and last chapters can be a little shorter, which might give you another 300–500 words to play with.

THE CHAPTER STRUCTURE

We have already said quite a lot about the content of the first four chapters so we will only revisit them briefly here. We will, though, discuss the conclusion at more length, partly because this often seems to get written in a hurry and lets down the other elements of the dissertation. Remember what we just said about aiming for 4×17 marks rather than $3 \times 18 + 5$!

Background and problem statement

You will often find this described as the 'Introduction' because it is the chapter where you set up all the things you are going to do in the rest of the dissertation. In Chapter 3, we suggested that you should write a problem statement to summarise your work up to that point. This should be the basis for the first chapter of the dissertation. How did you decide to study this topic – from your clinical experience, from your course reading, from a media story or whatever? How did you work through the process of turning this into a research question? How do you plan to answer that question in the following chapters? Is there a need for this to be investigated? If it has been investigated, is there a weakness in the resulting work?

Literature review

We described the Literature review in Chapter 4. Remember our metaphor of the wall. What does that wall look like? Where is the hole you are going to fill – or the weak point you are going to strengthen? What shape is it? How could it best be filled?

Justification and description of methods

This draws on the work you did in Chapters 5 to 8. This is where you explain why your project is an appropriate way to achieve the objective you identified in the Literature review and describe what you actually did, including your concern to carry out the work in an ethical way. We think you can best use this space if you do not spend too much time criticising the methods you did not choose rather than demonstrating how your approach was a logical way to answer your question and add to (and what was missing from) previous studies. It is easy in qualitative essays to be too critical of quantitative methods, for example, by suggesting that they cannot deal with problems they are not designed to deal with or that they think about knowledge and facts in ways that are radically different from those used in qualitative research. These are complex issues and you risk sounding very naïve about them, which does not help with getting a good mark from many supervisors. Accentuate the positive. Show why your approach is right rather than dismissing others as necessarily wrong.

> ## Key Point
>
> Do not forget what we said in Chapter 5 about there being more to ethics than getting the approval of an ethics review panel. Your department will probably expect you to declare somewhere in the dissertation that it has received ethics approval, but you should also discuss what made your data collection ethical.

—————————————— **VIDEO SUPPORT** ——————————————

It may be helpful at this stage to watch *Writing Up Social Research: Part 2 of 3 on Practical Issues and Ethics*, which, using role-play and interviews with experts, explores the ethical dilemmas that must be considered when doing research. You can access the video by visiting this book's online resources: https://study.sagepub.com/dingwallandstaniland.

Discussion and analysis of data

This is sometimes described as the 'Findings' chapter, but qualitative researchers are often uncomfortable with this label. 'Findings' can imply a degree of certainty that is hard to achieve with one small-scale and individual piece of research unless it is very closely integrated with previous studies. If, however, it is the language that your department prefers, you should use it. The chapter will be based on the work you did in Chapters 6 to 9. It is where you lay out what you saw, heard or read, or even sometimes what you smelled, and explain its significance to the reader.

Key Point

Remember that you are being marked on what is in the dissertation and that your marker is not telepathic! If something is not on the page or the screen, it does not exist, and you cannot get any credit for it. Remember that often in supervision sessions a student can explain a point very clearly but needs to be prompted that it would be better put on paper, rather than stay in their head. If you use a quote from a fieldnote, an interview or a document, you must explain what it means and why it matters. Never just insert a data extract and assume that the reader will make sense of it in the same way that you do. Nor should you insert the extract and write 'as we can see from this extract, X is the case'; point to specific words, phrases or actions that justify your inference, so the markers can follow your reasoning and check it for themselves.

We turn now to an important point to mention in academic research, that of *plagiarism*. Simply put, plagiarism involves taking the work of another person and using it as if it were one's own. The source of the original material is hidden, by not referencing it properly or by paraphrasing it without acknowledgement, or by not mentioning it at all. Plagiarism may occur in all forms of assessment, including written examinations. There are different types of plagiarism:

Definitions

Self-plagiarism (or double submission) is submitting work on two or more occasions (without proper acknowledgement) for separate credit. This may include the re-use of text, research data and so on without specific reference. It does not, however, normally include work submitted for reassessment or retake.

Collusion occurs when two or more students collaborate in the preparation and production of work which is submitted as the product of their individual efforts. Be aware that one student allowing another to use their own work is considered an act of collusion by both parties, regardless of intent.

Falsifying experimental or other investigative results that make it appear that information has been collected by scientific investigation, the compilation of results and so on, where it has actually been made up or edited to remove data that do not fit with the preferred findings.

Key Point

Research is a major part of university education, and it is expected that you will read, understand and discuss the writings of others. When writing your assignments, you will refer to existing literature on your subject, such as books, journals, online dissertations, newspapers, social media and websites. It is essential that you learn how to reference correctly, so you can acknowledge the contribution that others have made to your own work, provide evidence for your statements, and protect yourself against accusations of plagiarism. It is very important that you refer to the relevant institutional policy on referencing and plagiarism, understand and follow the policy. There are many online resources which introduce how to paraphrase, summarise, quote, in-text cite and reference in order to avoid plagiarism and achieve better marks.

Writing a conclusion

This task gets a section all to itself because its importance is often overlooked, which means that it gains fewer marks than it should do. The Conclusion is where everything comes together, so it looks backward over the whole dissertation. However, a good conclusion also looks forward to the next case study – or the next brick for the wall!

The first thing to do is to look again at the Introduction. What have you said you were going to do? Have you done that? If not, you may want to revise the Introduction so that it matches what you have done. Alternatively, you may want to begin the Conclusion by putting your hands up and saying, 'I know I said I would do *this*, but actually I have done *that*'. Of course, you then need to explain why you have not been able to deliver what you promised. Perhaps the people you were studying were unco-operative or they thought that other problems were more important or the way they worked and related to each other was not quite what you expected. There is nothing wrong with failing to achieve your original objectives as long as you can explain why and show that you have learned how you would do the project differently next time. What you absolutely must do, though, is to avoid having a beginning and an ending that do not match and give no explanation for this. This is one of the commonest mistakes at all academic levels.

——————————— VIDEO SUPPORT ———————————

If you are struggling with this, the video *Results, Discussion, Conclusion Chapters* offers some useful guidance on the writing of the final chapters within a dissertation. You can access the video by visiting this book's online resources: https://study.sagepub.com/dingwallandstaniland.

When you are clear about the relationship between the Introduction and the Conclusion, you should begin by summarising what you actually did, how you did it and what you learned (or found) from it. You do not need to allocate much space to this – it is simply a reminder to your reader about what has been important in the dissertation so far. This is not the place to justify what you did, either in your choice of methods or in the model you adopted for the research. Focus on the positive. Of course, you have done some good work and found interesting things – you do not need to worry about what you might have missed or done differently at this point. As you write this summary, you should be thinking about how you can link your case study to your wider reading. Does it look like something you referred to in the literature review? Does it look different? Can you explain why? Can you translate your observations into a more general, theoretical, language that will relate them to the work of other people? This is more important for Master's and PhD dissertations, but even undergraduates should be able to show how their particular study relates to books or articles that they have read.

 These connections are important for two reasons. First, they allow you to make reasonable criticisms of your own work. Many departments expect the conclusion to include a section that discusses the strengths and weaknesses of the study. This is a way for them to evaluate what you have learned from doing this exercise. In our experience, though, many students end up exaggerating the weaknesses of their own work by emphasising its small scale, limited time, single site, use of a single method and similar flaws. These may be true, but why give too much ammunition to your readers? If you can show that, despite the constraints of time, resources, access and what ethics regulators will allow, you have produced a study that fits with the existing literature, either to support it or to raise questions about it, then you can make a good case for its overall value.

The strength of a wall does not come from individual bricks but from the bonds between them. Of course, you cannot claim to have changed the entire world with a single study – but do not set out to trash your own work!

The second reason for making connections is to provide more support for any recommendations that you want to make for policy or practice. As we stressed in the early chapters, the point of nursing research is to make a difference. You want patients to be treated more nicely or more fairly. You want the health service to work more efficiently or effectively, so that its resources are not wasted doing the wrong things or the right things in the wrong way. As a small, one-off piece of work, you are unlikely to make much impact. However, if you can show that there is a body of research that is pointing in a particular direction – and you have now added to that – you can justify your recommendations more strongly. Suppose you have been looking at the way nurses talk to patients and whether this promotes patient dignity. There are published studies from the US, Canada, Australia and some of the Nordic countries to show that nurses use particular kinds of language that are not particularly professional and tend to infantilize their patients. Your observations are then a way to show 'it is happening all over – and it happens here too!'.

When making recommendations, it is important not to assume that there is only one solution to a problem or that your findings only point in one direction. Research is intended to inform the decisions that people with responsibility for policy or practice actually have to make. They may have to weigh research findings against other considerations. If they have a fixed budget, for example, your work may suggest that they would get better value by doing more for patient group X, but they would have to reduce service to patient group Y, which is well organised, articulate, and has a hotline to the local news media. You might think that this was an improper consideration, but the manager involved has to think about how the service is seen more generally and how this might affect its ability to get the resources that it needs to work at all. Your recommendations should also be closely connected to your research. Remember our earlier warnings about thinking that you should do qualitative research just to illustrate something that 'everybody knows' already. Your dissertation is probably not the place to argue for a complete reconstruction of the nursing profession and its relationship to global capitalism.

Finally, many departments like a Conclusion to finish with suggestions for further research. Again, it is important not to undermine what you have already done. How could it be built on? What might the next student's dissertation look like? If you have been doing fieldwork on a particular speciality ward, what other speciality wards might be good places to check out how far your findings can be generalised? Which might be similar? Which might be different in ways that would challenge your conclusions? In Chapter 2, for example, we described a number of studies of patient management in A&E departments. These showed some broad similarities between the UK, the US, and France – but also suggested that the process can work differently between university-affiliated hospitals and local general hospitals. Nurses often play a bigger role in the latter because many of the doctors working there are lower-status within their own profession. If we think about how nurses talk to patients, is this different in wards with a lot of longer-stay elderly patients than wards with a rapid throughput of younger and more articulate patients?

POLISHING YOUR WRITING

We thought we should finish this chapter with some suggestions about what makes for good writing in the context of a dissertation, and how to make your own writing better. These are just suggestions because writing style is quite a personal thing and your supervisor or department may also have their own preferences. However, our thoughts may help you to reflect on what you are doing. Even if you do not agree with us, it can be helpful to define why you do not agree.

1   *Look for good models.* Every time you read a book, a magazine, a blog or a newspaper, ask yourself whether you think it is well or badly written. What makes you want to read the next sentence or the next paragraph — or makes you think it is boring, pretentious or pompous? Social research writing is not the same as journalism or fiction writing, but you can learn a lot from those styles. Journalists and novelists make their living from capturing and holding the attention of their readers. What holds your attention? What loses it? Look particularly at the headline to an article, which is generally the key — does it make you want to read more?

2   *Short words are usually better than long ones,* unless you need to use a technical term. You do not make yourself look cleverer by picking obscure words out of the thesaurus on MS Word.

3   *Short sentences* are usually better than long ones.

4   *Do not forget to use paragraphs.* If you find a paragraph is much longer than 250 words, ask yourself whether you are trying to get too many ideas into one place. There is no need to be mechanical about this: paragraph lengths can vary and make the text more interesting. Just be sure that long ones are justified.

5   *Dissertations require reasonably formal writing and grammar.* Avoid street language, unless, of course, it is in the quotes from your informants!

6   *Be sure you know the difference between:* compliment and complement; discrete and discreet; disinterested and uninterested; affect and effect; elicit and illicit; infer and imply; flaunt and flout; mitigate and militate; inquiry and enquiry; ensure and insure; grisly and grizzly; practice and practise; principal and principle; program and programme.

7   *Don't try to write too much at one session.* Take regular breaks. These allow your mind to relax and refresh. When you come back, you will more easily see what you need to do next.

8   *Use the Speak/Read Aloud function in MS Word* to check your style — and help with your proof-reading. One of the easiest ways to spot sentences that are too long and complicated is to read them aloud — we often do it to our students. If we run out of breath before the end of a sentence, it shows the student that they need to fix the sentence. MS Word does not run out of breath, but if you lose the will to live before the end of a sentence, that is a pretty good signal that something is wrong.

9   *Use active verbs when you can:* 'I saw', not the passive form 'it was observed'. Different disciplines have different expectations here so you may be required to use passive sentences. However, qualitative researchers are generally quite comfortable with admitting their own part in the research and it does make the writing livelier.

10 *Always remember who you are writing for* – your reader. You may be obliged to write; your reader is not obliged to read! More exactly, the examiners for your dissertation may be obliged to read it but they can do that with more or less good will. You want them to enjoy the experience and look positively on your efforts. Try to inject a little cheer into their otherwise miserable lives.

THE END IS NEAR …

We have done our best to set out our thoughts and share our experience about qualitative research. Even if you never do another research project, this one will have helped you with important skills for your career. You should have learned how to analyse problems and to break them down into manageable units. You will know how to find resources that might help you to solve them – or at least to reduce their impact. Through your fieldwork, you will have learned how to watch people, to ask questions and to listen to the answers. You should understand how documents are created in health care organisations, and how to decode them. Now you have brought all these skills together in a final report.

This is not just an academic exercise, though. All of these are skills you will need in practice. How can you walk into a ward, or a patient's home, and make rapid and accurate judgements from what you see around you? How can you ask patients relevant questions and sort out what is important about their answers? How are the answers affected by their desire to create a particular impression on you? Are they not feeling pain or are they trying to show how brave they are? When your employer sends round a new document about their strategy and your part in it, what are they really saying? What are they trying to achieve? Is there really anything new here or is it just new words for the same old practices? Are they concerned about quality improvement or saving money? Of course, if your career takes you into management or leadership positions, you will also have to create these documents yourself. You will have to deal with the challenge of constructing them in ways that their intended readers find clear and persuasive. Your dissertation should be the capstone on the first phase of your learning as a nurse – and the foundation for learning that will go on throughout your life as society, technology and health care organisations change and develop. This is your contribution to the future of your profession.

CHAPTER SUMMARY POINTS

This chapter has outlined some key points to consider when writing your dissertation. We have made some suggestions from our own experiences of supervision and from some of the problems our own students have had.

FURTHER READING

There are a number of useful books on the craft of writing. The first of these is more immediately practical but focused on essay writing. The second was produced from a writing workshop and is co-authored by one of the graduate students involved and the workshop leader, an experienced academic writer. It is more discursive but may also help you think more deeply about what you are doing. The books by Howard Becker that we recommended at the end of the previous chapter also contain useful material.

Coleman, H. (2020) *Polish Your Academic Writing*. London: Sage.

Balmer, A. and Murcott, A. (2017) *The Craft of Writing in Sociology*. Manchester: Manchester University Press.

These articles expand on the relationship between a student and their dissertation tutor or supervisor and on the ways in which a qualitative dissertation might be assessed:

Turner, G.W. and Crane, B. (2016) 'Teaching and learning qualitative methods through the dissertation advising relationship: perspectives from a professor and a graduate', *Qualitative Social Work*, 15(3): 346–62. Available at https://doi.org/10.1177/1473325015626260 (accessed 29/2/20).

Peterson, J.S. (2019) 'Presenting a qualitative study: a reviewer's perspective', *Gifted Child Quarterly*, 63(3): 147–58. Available at https://doi.org/10.1177/0016986219844789 (accessed 29/2/20).

Appendix

USEFUL DATABASES FOR LITERATURE REVIEWS

Key resources

Database	Resource
NHS Evidence	This database searches a limited number of high-quality sources.
TRIP database	This database searches a limited number of high-quality sources.
Cochrane Library	This is the main source of systematic reviews in health care.
Royal Marsden Manual of Clinical Nursing Procedures	This database is a key resource for over 350 evidence-based clinical procedures related to every aspect of practical care.

General databases

Database	Resource
Pubmed Medline Emcare	A good starting point for any health or medical literature search.
CINAHL	Primary source of nursing and allied health literature.
BNI	British Nursing Index – resource for nursing literature.
PsycINFO	A resource for psychology and psychiatry literature.
Global Health	A resource of public health literature.

Multi-disciplinary

Database	Resource
Science Direct	A leading source for scientific, technical and medical research. Explore journals, books and articles.
Web of Science	Multi-disciplinary database, including links to Citation Indexes (citing articles) and Journal Impact Factors.
Scopus	Multi-disciplinary database, including links to citing articles.
Applied Social Sciences Index and Abstracts (ASSIA)	Multi-disciplinary social sciences database.

Subject specific

Database	Resource
Health Business Elite	Resource for health care administration.
HMIC	Health Information Management Consortium – great information from Department of Health and King's Fund.
AMED	Allied and Complementary Medicine Database.
PEDro	Physiotherapy Evidence Database.
OTSeeker	Searches systematic reviews and randomised controlled trials relevant to occupational therapy.
Educational Resources Information Center (ERIC)	Useful database on education research.

It may also be useful to note that many social scientists prefer Google Scholar, which is freely available and very easy to use. Librarians are often critical of Google Scholar, which is less selective in its content and may return less rigorous work in search results. However, it has much better coverage of books and book chapters. These are important in the social sciences but tend to be excluded by other databases. For qualitative research in health care, you may also find it useful to know about EQUATOR Network – this Library contains a comprehensive searchable database of reporting guidelines and also links to other resources relevant to research reporting at www.equator-network.org and the National Institute for Clinical Excellence (NICE) at www. evidence.nhs.uk.

References

Allen, D. (1998) 'Record-keeping and routine nursing practice: the view from the wards', *Journal of Advanced Nursing*, 27(6): 1223–30. Available at https://doi.org/10.1046/j.1365-2648.1998.00645.x (accessed 24/2/20).

Allen, D. (2002) *The Changing Shape of Nursing Practice: The Role of Nurses in the Hospital Division of Labour*. London: Routledge.

Allen, D. (2014a) *The Invisible Work of Nurses: Hospitals, Organisation and Healthcare*. London: Routledge.

Allen, D. (2014b) 'Lost in translation? "Evidence" and the articulation of institutional logics in integrated care pathways: from positive to negative boundary object?', *Sociology of Health & Illness*, 36(6): 807–22. Available at https://onlinelibrary.wiley.com/doi/full/10.1111/1467-9566.12111 (accessed 24/2/20).

Ashley, J. and Stamp K. (2014) 'Learning to think like a nurse: the development of clinical judgment in nursing students', *Journal of Nursing Education*, 53(9): 519–25. Available at www.ncbi.nlm.nih.gov/pubmed/25199107 (accessed 24/2/20).

Atkinson, P. and Coffey, A. (1997) 'Analysing documentary realities', in D. Silverman (ed.), *Qualitative Research: Theory, Methods and Practice*. London: Sage. pp. 44–62.

Atkinson, P. and Silverman, D. (1997) 'Kundera's Immortality: The interview society and the invention of the self', *Qualitative Inquiry*, 3(3): 304–325. Available at https://doi.org/10.1177/107780049700300304 (accessed 24/3/20).

Balmer, A. and Murcott, A. (2017) *The Craft of Writing in Sociology*. Manchester: Manchester University Press.

Banks, M. and Zeitlyn, D. (2015) *Visual Methods in Social Research* (2nd edn). London: Sage.

Barnett-Page, E. and Thomas, J. (2009) 'Methods for the synthesis of qualitative research: a critical review', *BMC Medical Research Methodology*, 9(1): 59. Available at https://bmcmedresmethodol.biomedcentral.com/articles/10.1186/1471-2288-9-59 (accessed 24/2/20).

Beauchamp, T. and Childress, J. (2019) *Principles of Biomedical Ethics* (8th edn). New York: Oxford University Press.

Becker, H.S. (1998) *Tricks of the Trade: How to Think about Your Research while You're Doing It*. Chicago, IL: University of Chicago Press.

Becker, H.S. (2007) *Telling About Society*. Chicago, IL: University of Chicago Press.

Becker, H.S. (2017) *Evidence*. Chicago, IL: University of Chicago Press.

Berg, B.L. (2007) *Qualitative Research Methods for the Social Sciences* (6th edn). London: Pearson.

Bircumshaw, D. (1990) 'The utilization of research findings in clinical nursing practice', *Journal of Advanced Nursing*, 15(11): 1272–80. Available at https://doi.org/10.1111/j.1365-2648.1990.tb01742.x (accessed 24/2/20).

Bloch, S. and Leydon, G. (2019) 'Conversation analysis and telephone helplines for health and illness: a narrative review', *Research on Language and Social Interaction*, 52(3): 193–211. Available at https://doi.org/10.1080/08351813.2019.1631035 (accessed 24/32/20).

Bloor, M.J, Frankland, J., Thomas, M. and Robson, K. (2000) *Focus Groups in Social Research*. London: Sage.

Bolton, R. (1995) 'Tricks, friends and lovers: erotic encounters in the field', in D. Kulick and M. Willson (eds), *Taboo: Sex, Identity and Erotic Subjectivity in Anthropological Fieldwork*. London: Routledge. pp. 140–67.

Boore, J.R.P. (1978) *Prescription for Recovery*. London: Royal College of Nursing.

Booth, W.C., Colomb, G.C., Williams, J.M., Bizup, H. and Fitzgerald, W.T. (2016) *The Craft of Research* (4th edn). Chicago, IL: University of Chicago Press.

Boswell, J. (2008 [1791]) *The Life of Samuel Johnson*. London: Penguin Classics.

Bourgeault, I., Dingwall, R. and de Vries, R.G. (eds) (2010) *Qualitative Methods in Health Research*. London: Sage.

Bowen, G. (2009) 'Document analysis as a qualitative research method', *Qualitative Research Journal*, 9(2): 27–40. Available at https://doi.org/10.3316/qrj0902027 (accessed 24/2/20).

Bowler, I. (1993) '"They're not the same as us": midwives' stereotypes of South Asian descent maternity patients', *Sociology of Health & Illness*, 15(2): 157–78. Available at https://onlinelibrary.wiley.com/doi/abs/10.1111/1467-9566.ep11346882 (accessed 24/2/20).

Briggs, A. (1972) *Report of the Committee on Nursing*. Cmnd 5115. London: HMSO.

Britt, R. and Englebert, A. (2019) 'Experiences of patients living with inflammatory bowel disease in rural communities', *Qualitative Research in Medicine and Healthcare*, 3(1): 40–6. Available at https://doi.org/10.4081/qrmh.2019.7962 (accessed 24/2/20).

Britten, N., Campbell, R., Pope, C., Donovan, J., Morgan, M. and Pill, R. (2002) 'Using meta ethnography to synthesise qualitative research: a worked example', *Journal of Health Services Research & Policy*, 7(4): 209–15. Available at https://doi.org/10.1258/135581902320432732 (accessed 24/2/20).

Burgess, R.G. (1984) *In the Field: An Introduction to Field Research*. London: HarperCollins.

Campbell, R., Pound, P., Morgan, M., Daker-White, G., Britten, N., Pill, R., Yardley, L., Pope, C. and Donovan, J. (2011) 'Evaluating meta ethnography: systematic analysis and synthesis of qualitative research', *Health Technology Assessment*, 15(43). Available at https://doi.org/10.3310/hta15430 (accessed 24/2/20).

Cappelletti, A., Engel, J.K. and Prentice, D. (2014) 'Systematic review of clinical judgment and reasoning in nursing', *Journal of Nursing Education*, 53(8):453–8. Available at https://doi.org/10.3928/01484834-20140724-01 (accessed 24/2/20).

Chen, S-L.S., Chen, Z.J. and Allaire, N. (2019) *Building Sexual Misconduct Cases against Powerful Men*. Lanham, MD: Lexington Books.

Cohen, W.M. and Levinthal, D.A. (1990) 'Absorptive capacity: a new perspective on learning and innovation', *Administrative Science Quarterly*, 35(1): 128–52. Available at https://doi.org/10.2307/2393553 (accessed 24/2/20).

Coleman, H. (2020) *Polish Your Academic Writing*. London: Sage.

Cooke, C., Smith, A. and Booth, A. (2012) 'Beyond PICO: The SPIDER tool for qualitative evidence synthesis', *Qualitative Health Research*, 22(10):1435–43. Available at https://doi.org/10.1177/1049732312452938 (accessed 24/2/20).

Coughlan, M. and Cronin, P. (2016) *Doing a Literature Review in Nursing, Health and Social Care* (2nd edn). London: Sage.

Cranley L., Doran, D.M., Tourangeau, A.E., Kushniruk, A. and Nagle, L.(2009) 'Nurses' uncertainty in decision-making: a literature review', *Worldviews on Evidence-Based Nursing*,6(1): 3–15. Available at https://doi.org/10.1111/j.1741-6787.2008.00138.x (accessed 24/2/20).

Critical Appraisal Skills Programme (CASP) (2017) '10 questions to help you make sense of qualitative research'. Available at http://docs.wixstatic.com/ugd/dded87_25658615020e427da194a325e7773d42.pdf (accessed 26/2/20).

Critical Appraisal Skills Programme *CASP* (CASP Checklist) (2018) available at https://casp-uk.net/wp-content/uploads/2018/01/CASP-Qualitative-Checklist-2018.pdf (accessed 07/05/2020).

Critical Appraisal Skills Programme UK. (n.d.). CASP checklists. Retrieved from https://casp-uk.net/casp-tools-checklists/

Depape, A-M. and Lindsay, S. (2015) 'Parents' experiences of caring for a child with autism spectrum disorder', *Qualitative Health Research*, 25(4): 569–83. Available at https://doi.org/10.1177/1049732314552455 (accessed 24/2/20).

Department of Health (1999) *Making a Difference: Strengthening the Nursing, Midwifery and Health Visiting Contribution to Health and Social Care.* London: HMSO. Available at http://webarchive.nationalarchives.gov.uk/20130107105354/http://www.dh.gov.uk/prod_consum_dh/groups/dh_digitalassets/@dh/@en/documents/digitalasset/dh_4074704.pdf (accessed 18/9/19).

Department of Health (2011) *Front Line Care: The Report of the Prime Minister's Commission on the Future of Nursing and Midwifery in England.* Available at http://webarchive.nationalarchives.gov.uk/20100331110400/http:/cnm.independent.gov.uk/wp-content/uploads/2010/03/front_line_care.pdf (accessed 18/9/19).

Department of Health (2012) *Developing the Role of the Clinical Academic Researcher in the Nursing, Midwifery and Allied Health Professions.* Available at www.gov.uk/government/publications/developing-the-role-of-the-clinical-academic-researcher-in-the-nursing-midwifery-and-allied-health-professions (accessed 18/9/19).

DeWalt, K.M. and DeWalt, B.R. (2010) *Participant Observation: A Guide for Fieldworkers* (2nd edn). Lanham, MD: Rowman Altamira.

Dingwall, R. (1974) 'Some sociological aspects of "nursing research"', *Sociological Review*, 22(1): 45–55. https://journals.sagepub.com/doi/abs/10.1111/j.1467-954X.1974.tb00241.x (accessed 24/2/20).

Dingwall, R. (1977) *The Social Organisation of Health Visitor Training.* London: Croom Helm.

Dingwall, R. (1980) 'Ethics and ethnography', *Sociological Review*, 28(4): 871–91. Available at https://doi.org/10.1111/j.1467-954x.1980.tb00599.x (accessed 24/2/20).

Dingwall, R. (1992) 'Don't mind him – he's from Barcelona: qualitative methods in health studies', in J. Daly, I. McDonald and E. Willis (eds), *Researching Health Care.* London: Routledge. pp. 161–75.

Dingwall, R. (1997) 'Accounts, interviews and observations,' in G. Miller and R. Dingwall (eds), *Context and Method in Qualitative Research.* London: Sage. pp. 51–65.

Dingwall, R. (2008) *Qualitative Health Research* (4 vols). London: Sage.

Dingwall, R. and Allen, D. (2001) 'The implications of healthcare reforms for the profession of nursing', *Nursing Inquiry* 8(2): 64–74. Available at https://doi.org/10.1046/j.1440-1800.2001.00100.x (accessed 24/2/20).

Dingwall, R. and Murray, T. (1983) 'Categorization in accident departments: "good" patients, "bad" patients and "children"', *Sociology of Health & Illness*, 5(2): 127–48. Available at https://onlinelibrary.wiley.com/doi/pdf/10.1111/1467-9566.ep10491496 (accessed 24/2/20).

Dingwall, R., Eekeleaar, J. and Murray, T. (2014) *The Protection of Children: State Intervention and Family Life* (2nd edn). New Orleans, LA: Quid Pro Books.

Dingwall, R., Murphy, E., Watson, P., Greatbatch, D. and Parker, S. (1998) 'Catching goldfish: quality in qualitative research', *Journal of Health Services Research and Policy*, 3(3): 167–72. Available at https://doi.org/10.1177/135581969800300308 (accessed 24/2/20).

Dingwall, R., Rafferty, A.M. and Webster, C. (1988) *An Introduction to the Social History of Nursing*. London: Routledge.

Dingwall, R., Tanaka, H. and Minamikata, S. (1991) 'Images of parenthood in the United Kingdom and Japan', *Sociology*, 25(3): 423–46. Available at https://doi.org/10.1177/0038038591025003005 (accessed 24/2/20).

Dodier, N. and Camus, A. (1998) 'Openness and specialisation: dealing with patients in a hospital emergency service', *Sociology of Health & Illness*, 20(4): 413–44. Available at https://doi.org/10.1111/1467-9566.00109 (accessed 24/2/20).

Emerson, R.M., Fretz, R I. and Shaw, L.L. (2011) *Writing Ethnographic Fieldnotes* (2nd edn). Chicago, IL: University of Chicago Press.

Emmison, M., Smith, P. and Mayall, M. (2012) *Researching the Visual*. London: Sage.

Flemming, K. and Briggs, M. (2007) 'Electronic searching to locate qualitative research: evaluation of three strategies', *Journal of Advanced Nursing*, 57(1): 95–100. Available at https://doi.org/10.1111/j.1365-2648.2006.04083.x (accessed 24/2/20).

Francis, R. (2013) *Report of the Mid Staffordshire NHS Foundation Trust Public Inquiry* (HC 947). London: The Stationery Office.

French, P. (2002) 'What is the evidence on evidence-based nursing? An epistemological concern', *Journal of Advanced Nursing*, 37(3): 250–57. Available at https://doi.org/10.1046/j.1365-2648.2002.02065.x (accessed 24/2/20).

Friedman, N. (1967) *The Social Nature of Psychological Research: The Psychological Experiment as a Social Interaction*. Oxford: Basic Books.

Garcia, A.C. (2013) *An Introduction to Interaction: Understanding Talk in Formal and Informal Settings*. London: Bloomsbury.

Garfinkel, H. (1967) *Studies in Ethnomethodology*. Englewood Cliffs, N.J.: Prentice-Hall.

Gerth, H.H. and Wright Mills, C., eds (1970) *From Max Weber*. London: Routledge & Kegan Paul.

Gold, R. (1958) 'Roles in sociological field observation', *Social Forces*, 36(3): 217–13. Available at https://doi.org/10.2307/2573808 (accessed 24/2/20).

Goodwin, C. (1994) 'Professional vision,' *American Anthropologist*, 96(3): 606–633. Available at https://doi.org/10.1525/aa.1994.96.3.02a00100 (accessed 24/2/20).

Hale, R. (2016) *'An actor-network analysis of the healthcare worker influenza immunisation programme in Wales, 2009–2011'*. PhD thesis, University of Nottingham.

Hammersley, M. and Atkinson, P. (2019) *Ethnography: Principles in Practice* (4th edn). London: Routledge.

Harper, R.H., O'Hara, K.P., Sellen, A.J. and Duthie, D.J. (1997) 'Toward the paperless hospital?', *British Journal of Anaesthesia*, 78(6): 762–67. Available at https://doi.org/10.1093/bja/78.6.762 (accessed 24/2/20).

Hart, C. (2018) *Doing a Literature Review: Releasing the Research Imagination*. London: Sage.

Hayward, J. (1975) *Information – A prescription against pain*. London: Royal College of Nursing.

Hedgecoe, A. (2014) 'A deviation from standard design? Clinical trials, research ethics committees, and the regulatory co-construction of organizational deviance', *Social Studies of Science*, 44(1): 59–81. Available at https://doi.org/10.1177/0306312713506141 (accessed 24/2/20).

Hills, T., Proto, E., Sgroi, D. and Seresinhe, C.I. (2019) 'Historical analysis of national subjective wellbeing using millions of digitized books', *Nature Human Behaviour*, 3: 1271–5. Available at https://doi.org/10.1038/s41562-019-0750-z (accessed 24/2/20).

Hochschild, A.R. (1983) *The Managed Heart: Commercialization of Human Feeling*. Berkeley, CA: University of California Press.

Hollis, M. (2002). *The Philosophy of Social Science: An Introduction* (Revised edn). Cambridge: Cambridge University Press.

Hughes, D. (1980) *'Lay assessment of clinical seriousness: practical decision-making by non-medical staff in a hospital Casualty Department'*. PhD thesis, University of Wales, Swansea.

Hughes, D. (2018) 'Informed consent, judicial review and the uncertainties of ethnographic research in sensitive NHS settings', *Sage Research Methods Cases* (Online Collection). London: Sage. Available at https://cronfa.swan.ac.uk/Record/cronfa33668 doi: 10.4135/9781526431561 (accessed 24/2/20).

Hughes, R. (1998) 'Considering the vignette technique and its application to a study of drug injecting and HIV risk and safer behaviour', *Sociology of Health & Illness,* 20(3): 381–400. Available at https://doi.org/10.1111/1467-9566.00107 (accessed 24/2/20).

Hull, E. (2017) *Contingent Citizens: Professional Aspiration in a South African Hospital.* London: Bloomsbury.

Israel, M. (2014) *Research Ethics and Integrity for Social Scientists: Beyond Regulatory Compliance* (2nd edn). London: Sage.

Jeffery, R. (1979) 'Normal rubbish: deviant patients in casualty departments', *Sociology of Health & Illness,* 1(1): 90–107. Available at https://doi.org/10.1111/1467-9566.ep11006793 (accessed 24/2/20).

Johannessen, L.E. (2019) 'Negotiated discretion: redressing the neglect of negotiation in "street-level bureaucracy"', *Symbolic Interaction,* 42(4). Available at https://doi.org/10.1002/symb.451 (accessed 24/2/20).

Kara, H. (2017) *Creative Research Methods in the Social Sciences: A Practical Guide.* Bristol: Policy Press.

Kara, H. (2018) *Research Ethics in the Real World: Euro-Western and Indigenous Perspectives.* Bristol: Policy Press.

Kim, E-K., Park, E.Y., Gong, J-W.S., Jang, S-H., Choi, Y-H. and Lee, H-K. (2017) 'Lasting effect of an oral hygiene care program for patients with stroke during in-hospital rehabilitation: a randomized single-center clinical trial', *Disability and Rehabilitation,* 39(22): 2324–9. Available at https://doi.org/10.1080/09638288.2016.1226970 (accessed 24/2/20).

Lenette, C., Cox, L. and Brough, M. (2015) 'Digital storytelling as a social work tool: learning from ethnographic research with women from refugee backgrounds', *British Journal of Social Work,* 45(3): 988–1005. Available at http://dx.doi.org/10.1093/bjsw/bct184 (accessed 24/2/20).

Lindesmith, A.R. (1965) *The Addict and the Law.* Bloomington, IN: Indiana University Press.

Livingston, G., Kelly, L., Lewis-Holmes, E., Baio, G., Morris, S., Patel, N. and Cooper, C. (2014) 'A systematic review of the clinical effectiveness and cost-effectiveness of sensory, psychological and behavioural interventions for managing agitation in older adults with dementia', *Health Technology Assessment,* 18(39). Available at www.ncbi.nlm.nih.gov/pubmed/24947468 (accessed 24/2/20).

Loseke, D. (2016) *Methodological Thinking: Basic Principles of Social Research Design* (2nd edn). Thousand Oaks, CA: Sage.

Loseke, D. (2017) *Thinking about Social Problems: An Introduction to Constructionist Perspectives.* New York: Routledge.

Lune, H. and Berg, B.L. (2017) *Qualitative Research Methods for the Social Sciences* (9th edn). Harlow: Pearson.

Macintyre, S. (1978) 'Some notes on record taking and making in an antenatal clinic', *The Sociological Review,* 26(3): 595–612. Available at https://doi.org/10.1111/j.1467-954x.1978.tb00147.x (accessed 24/2/20).

Magnussen, I-L., Alteren, J. and Bondas, T. (2019) 'Appreciative inquiry in a Norwegian nursing home: a unifying and maturing process to forward new knowledge and new practice', *International Journal of Qualitative Studies on Health and Well-being,* 14(1). Available at www.tandfonline.com/doi/full/10.1080/17482631.2018.1559437 (accessed 24/2/20).

Malinowski, B. (1922) *Argonauts of the Western Pacific: An Account of Native Enterprise and Adventure in the Archipelagoes of Melanesian New Guinea*. London: Routledge. Available at www.gutenberg.org/ebooks/ 55822 (accessed 19/9/19).

McCaffery, M. and Beebe, A. (1989) *Pain: Clinical Manual for Nursing Practice*. St Louis, MO: C.V. Mosby.

McCrae, N. (2012) 'Whither nursing models? The value of nursing theory in the context of evidence-based practice and multidisciplinary health care', *Journal of Advanced Nursing*, 68(1): 222–9. https://onlinelibrary. wiley.com/doi/abs/10.1111/j.1365-2648.2011.05821.x (accessed 24/2/20).

McDonald, L. (2014) *Mary Seacole: The Making of the Myth*. Toronto: Iguana Books.

McDonald, L. (2019) 'The first BME nurse in the NHS'. Available at http://blogs.nottingham.ac.uk/ florencenightingale/2019/05/16/the-first-bme-nurse-in-the-nhs-by-professor-lynn-mcdonald/ (accessed 20/9/19).

Melia, K. (1987) *Learning and Working: The Occupational Socialization of Nurses*. London: Tavistock.

Meluch, A. (2018) 'Above and beyond: an exploratory study of breast cancer patient accounts of healthcare provider information-giving practices and informational support', *Qualitative Research in Medicine and Healthcare*, 2(2): 113–20. Available at https://doi.org/10.4081/qrmh.2018.7387 (accessed 24/2/20).

Menzies, I.E.P. (1960) 'A case-study in the functioning of social systems as a defence against anxiety: a report on a study of the nursing service of a general hospital', *Human Relations*, 13(2): 95–121. Available at https://doi.org/10.1177/001872676001300201 (accessed 24/2/20).

Merner, B., Hill, S. and Taylor, M. (2019) '"I'm trying to stop things before they happen": Carers' contributions to patient safety in hospitals', *Qualitative Health Research*, 29(10): 1508–18. Available at https://doi. org/10.1177/1049732319841021 (accessed 24/2/20).

Merton, R.K. (1995) 'The Thomas Theorem and the Matthew Effect', *Social Forces*, 74(2): 379–424. Available at https://doi.org/10.1093/sf/74.2.379 (accessed 24/2/20).

Methley, A.M., Campbell, S., Chew-Graham, C., McNally, R. and Cheraghi-Sohi, S. (2014) 'PICO, PICOS and SPIDER: a comparison study of specificity and sensitivity in three search tools for qualitative systematic reviews', *BMC Health Services Research*, 14: 579. Available at https://doi.org/10.1186/s12913- 014-0579-0 (accessed 24/2/20).

Mill, J.S. (1843) *A System of Logic*. New York: Harper & Bros.

Mondada, L. (2014) 'Instructions in the operating room: how the surgeon directs their assistant's hands,' *Discourse Studies*, 16(2): 131–61. Available at https://doi.org/10.1177/1461445613515325 (accessed 24/2/20).

Murphy, E. and Dingwall, R. (2001) 'The ethics of ethnography', in P. Atkinson, A. Coffey, S. Delamont, L. Lofland and J. Lofland (eds), *Handbook of Ethnography*. Sage: London. pp. 339–51.

Murphy, E. and Dingwall, R. (2003) *Qualitative Methods and Health Policy Research*. New York: Aldine de Gruyter.

Murphy, E., Dingwall, R., Greatbatch, D., Parker, S. and Watson, P. (1998) 'Qualitative research methods in health technology assessment: a review of the literature', *Health Technology Assessment*, 2(16). Available at https.doi.org/10.3310/hta2160 (accessed 10/05/20)

National Council of State Boards for Nursing (NCSBN) (2015) *Mission Statement Adopted by Delegate Assembly* (2010). Available at www.ncsbn.org/about.htm (accessed 22/10/19).

Newmahr, S. (2011) *Playing on the Edge: Sadomasochism, Risk, and Intimacy*. Bloomington, IN: Indiana University Press.

Nightingale, F. (1860) *Notes on Nursing: What it is, and What it is Not*. London: Harrison.

Noblitt, G. and Hare, R.D. (1988) *Meta-Ethnography: Synthesizing Qualitative Studies*. Sage University Paper series on Qualitative Research Methods, Volume 11. Beverley Hills, CA: Sage.

Nugus, P. (2019) 'Re-structuring the negotiated order of the hospital', *Sociology of Health & Illness*, 41(2): 378–94. https://onlinelibrary.wiley.com/doi/abs/10.1111/1467-9566.12838 (accessed 24/2/20).

Nursing and Midwifery Board of Australia (2018) *Midwife Standards for Practice*. Available at www.nursing-midwiferyboard.gov.au/Codes-Guidelines-Statements/Professional-standards/Midwife-standards-for-practice.aspx (accessed 21/1/20).

Nursing and Midwifery Council (2018a) *The Code: Professional Standards of Practice and Behaviour for Nurses, Midwives and Nursing Associates*. London: Nursing and Midwifery Council. Available at www.nmc.org.uk/standards/code/ (accessed 7/10/19).

Nursing and Midwifery Council (2018b) *Future Nurse: Standards of Proficiency for Registered Nurses*. London: Nursing and Midwifery Council. Available at www.nmc.org.uk/globalassets/sitedocuments/education-standards/future-nurse-proficiencies.pdf (accessed 19/9/19).

Oakley, A. (1998) 'Gender, methodology and people's ways of knowing: some problems with feminism and the paradigm debate in social science', *Sociology*, 32(4): 707–31.

Parry, R., Pino, M. and Faull, C. (2016) 'Acceptability and design of video-based research on healthcare communication: evidence and recommendations', *Patient Education and Counselling*, 99(8): 1271–84. Available at https://doi.org/10.1016/j.pec.2016.03.013 (accessed 24/2/20).

Pecanac, K.E. (2018) 'Combining conversation analysis and event sequencing to study health communication', *Research in Nursing & Health*, 41(3): 312–19. Available at https://doi.org/10.1002/nur.21863 (accessed 24/2/20).

Peterson, A.L. (2015) 'A case for the use of autoethnography in nursing research', *Journal of Advanced Nursing*, 71(1): 226–33. Available at https://doi.org/10.1111/jan.12501 (accessed 24/2/20).

Peterson, J.S. (2019) 'Presenting a qualitative study: a reviewer's perspective', *Gifted Child Quarterly*, 63(3): 147–58. Available at https://doi.org/10.1177/0016986219844789 (accessed 24/2/20).

Petticrew, M. and Roberts, H. (2008) *Systematic Reviews in the Social Sciences: A Practical Guide*. Oxford: Blackwell.

Pilnick, A. and Dingwall, R. (2011) 'On the remarkable persistence of asymmetry in doctor/patient interaction', *Social Science and Medicine*, 72(8): 1374–82. Available at https://doi.org/10.1016/j.socscimed.2011.02.033 (accessed 24/2/20).

Pink, S. and Morgan, J. (2013) 'Short-term ethnography: intense routes to knowing', *Symbolic Interaction*, 36(3): 351–61. Available at http://dx.doi.org/10.1002/symb.66 (accessed 24/2/20).

Preus, H.R., Maharajasingam, N., Rosic, J. and Baelum, V. (2019) 'Oral hygiene phase revisited: how different study designs have affected results in intervention studies', *Journal of Clinical Periodontology*, 46(5): 548–51. Available at https://doi.org/10.1111/jcpe.13109 (accessed 24/2/20).

Prior, L. (1989) *The Social Organisation of Death: Medical Discourse and Social Practices in Belfast*. London: Macmillan.

Prior, L. (2003) *Using Documents in Social Research*. London: Sage.

Reed, J. (1995) 'Practitioner knowledge in practitioner research', in J. Reed and S. Procter (eds), *Practitioner Research in Healthcare*. London: Chapman & Hall. pp 46–61.

Reich, J. (2016) *Calling the Shots: Why Parents Reject Vaccines*. New York: New York University Press.

Roth, J.A. (1957) 'Ritual and magic in the control of contagion', *American Sociological Review*, 22(3): 310–14. Available at https://doi.org/10.2307/2088472 (accessed 24/2/20).

Roth, J.A. (1972a) 'Some contingencies of the moral evaluation and control of clientele: the case of the hospital emergency service', *American Journal of Sociology*, 77(5): 839–56. Available at https://doi.org/10.1086/225227 (accessed 24/2/20).

Roth, J.A. (1972b) 'Staff and client control strategies in urban hospital emergency services', *Urban Life and Culture* (now *Journal of Contemporary Ethnography*), 1(1): 39–60. Available at https://doi.org/10.1177/089124167200100103 (accessed 24/2/20).

Rycroft-Malone, J., Harvey, J.G., Seers, K., Kitson, A., McCormack, B. and Titchen, A. (2004) 'An explanation of the factors that influence the implementation of evidence into practice', *Journal of Clinical Nursing*, 13(8): 913–24. Available at https://doi.org/10.1111/j.1365-2702.2004.01007.x (accessed 24/2/20).

Sbaih, L.C. (2002) 'Meanings of immediate: the practical use of the Patient's Charter in the accident and emergency department', *Social Science and Medicine*, 54(9): 1345–55. Available at https://doi.org/10.1016/s0277-9536(01)00100-9 (accessed 24/2/20).

Schwandt, T.A. (2015) *The SAGE Dictionary of Qualitative Inquiry* (4th edn). Thousand Oaks, CA: Sage.

Seacole, M. (2005) *Wonderful Adventures of Mrs Seacole in Many Lands.* London: Penguin.

Sellars, J. (2019) *Lessons in Stoicism: What Ancient Philosophers Teach Us about How to Live.* London: Allen Lane.

Sellen, A. and Harper, R. (2003) *The Myth of the Paperless Office.* Cambridge, MA: MIT Press.

Silver, C. and Lewins, A. (2014) *Using Software in Qualitative Research: A Step-by-Step Guide* (2nd edn). London: Sage.

Silverman, D. (2014) *Interpreting Qualitative Data* (5th edn). London: Sage.

Silverman, D. (2017) *Doing Qualitative Research* (5th edn). London: Sage.

Singer, P. and Kuhse, H. (1985) *Should the Baby Live? The Problem of Handicapped Infants.* Oxford: Oxford University Press.

Sointu, E. (2017) '"Good" patient/"bad" patient: clinical learning and the entrenching of inequality', *Sociology of Health & Illness*, 39(1): 63–77. Available at https://doi.org/10.1111/1467-9566.12487 (accessed 24/2/20).

Soyer, A. (1857) *Soyer's Culinary Campaign. Being Historical Reminiscences of the Late War. With The Plain Art of Cookery for Military and Civil Institutions, the Army, Navy, Public, Etc. Etc.* London: G. Routledge & Co. Available at www.gutenberg.org/ebooks/42544 (accessed 29/3/20).

Staniland, K.M. (2007) *Clinical Governance and Nursing: A Sociological Analysis.* PhD thesis, University of Salford, UK. Available at http://usir.salford.ac.uk/2062/1/Thesis_2008_Final_May_2009.pdf (accessed 7/10/19).

Stannard, C.I. (1973) 'Old folks and dirty work: the social conditions for patient abuse in a nursing home', *Social Problems*, 20(3): 329–42. Available at https://doi.org/10.2307/799597 (accessed 24/2/20).

Stockwell, F. (1972) *The Unpopular Patient.* London: Royal College of Nursing.

Stokoe, E. (2018) *Talk: The Science of Conversation.* London: Robinson

Strong, P.M. (2001) *The Ceremonial Order of the Clinic: Doctors, Patients and Medical Bureaucracies* (2nd edn). Aldershot: Ashgate.

Tajabadi, A., Ahmadi, F., Sadooghi Asl, A. and Vaismoradi, M. (2019) 'Unsafe nursing documentation: a qualitative content analysis', *Nursing Ethics.* Available at https://doi.org/10.1177%2F0969733019871682 (accessed 24/2/20).

ten Have, P. (2004) *Understanding Qualitative Research and Ethnomethodology.* London: Sage.

Thomas, R. (2019) *Turn Your Literature Review Into an Argument*: Little Quick Fix. London: Sage.

Thomas, W.I. and Thomas, D.S. (1928) *The Child in America.* New York: Alfred A. Knopf.

Thompson, W. (Lord Kelvin) (1883) 'Electrical units of measurement', in *Popular Lectures and Addresses.* London: Macmillan.

Toynbee, P. (2003) *Hard Work: Life in Low-pay Britain.* London: Bloomsbury.

Traynor, M. (1999) *Managerialism and Nursing.* London: Routledge.

Turner, G.W. and Crane, B. (2016) 'Teaching and learning qualitative methods through the dissertation advising relationship: perspectives from a professor and a graduate', *Qualitative Social Work*, 15(3): 346–62. Available at https://doi.org/10.1177/1473325015626260 (accessed 24/2/20).

United Nations (1948) *Universal Declaration of Human Rights*. Geneva: UN. Available at https://www.un.org/en/universal-declaration-human-rights/ (accessed 26/2/20).

Vassy, C. (2001) 'Categorisation and micro-rationing: access to care in a French emergency department', *Sociology of Health & Illness*, 23(5): 615–32. Available at https://doi.org/10.1111/1467-9566.00268 (accessed 24/2/20).

Viergever, R.F. (2019) 'The critical incident technique: method or methodology?', *Qualitative Health Research*, 29(7): 1065–79. Available at https://doi.org/10.1177/1049732318813112 (accessed 24/2/20).

vom Lehn, D. (2016) *Harold Garfinkel: The Creation and Development of Ethnomethodology*. Abingdon: Routledge.

Vuolo, J. (2014) 'In my lifetime – 30 years of nursing'. Available from http://lifetimenurse.blogspot.co.uk/2013_09_01_archive.html (accessed 19/9/19).

Walsh, M. and Ford, P. (1989) *Nursing Rituals, Research and Rational Action*. Oxford: Butterworth Heinemann.

Whittaker, E. and Olesen, V. (1964) 'The faces of Florence Nightingale: functions of the heroine legend in an occupational sub-culture', *Human Organization*, 23(2): 123–30. Available at https://doi.org/10.17730/humo.23.2.b555056w14706046 (accessed 24/2/20).

Wiener, C.L. (2000) *The Elusive Quest: Accountability in Hospitals*. New York: Aldine de Gruyter.

Williams, M. (2016) *Key Concepts in the Philosophy of Social Research*. London: Sage.

Witz, A. (1992) *Professions and Patriarchy*. London: Routledge.

World Health Organization. (2020) *WHO Director-General's opening remarks at the media briefing on COVID-19 – 11 March 2020*. Available at www.who.int/dg/speeches/detail/who-director-general-s-opening-remarks-at-the-media-briefing-on-covid-19---11-march-2020 (accessed 28/05/2020).

Wynn, L. and Israel, M. (2018) 'The fetishes of consent: signatures, paper, and writing in research ethics review', *American Anthropologist*, 120(4): 795–806.

Index